LANCHESTER LIBRARY

3 8001 00595 5293

Lanchester Library

WITHDRAWN

LANCHESTER LIBRARY, Coventry University
Gosford Street, Coventry CVI 5DD Telephone 024 7488

KT-472-326

Working with Children who need
Long-term Respiratory Support

Other Health & Social Care books from M&K include

The Management of COPD in Primary and Secondary Care
ISBN: 978-1-905539-28-4

Arterial Blood Gas Analysis: An easy learning guide
ISBN: 978-1-905539-04-8

The Clinician's Guide to Chronic Disease Management of Long-Term Conditions: A cognitive behaviour approach
ISBN: 978-1-905539-15-4

Paediatric Minor Emergencies
ISBN: 978-1-905539-35-2

Self-assessment in Paediatric Musculoskeletal Trauma X-rays
ISBN: 978-1-905539-34-5

Research Issues in Health and Social Care
ISBN: 978-1-905539-20-8

Nurses and Their Patients: Informing practice through psychodynamic insights
ISBN: 978-1-905539-31-4

Spiritual Assessment in Healthcare Practice
ISBN: 978-1-905539-27-7

Preoperative Assessment and Perioperative Management
ISBN: 978-1-905539-02-4

Ward-based Critical Care
ISBN: 978-1-905539-03-1

The ECG Workbook 2/e
ISBN: 978-1-905539-77-2

Working with Children who need Long-term Respiratory Support

Jaqui Hewitt-Taylor

Working with Children who need Long-term Respiratory Support
Jaqui Hewitt-Taylor

ISBN: 978-1-905539-69-7

First published 2011

All rights reserved. No part of this publication may be reproduced, stored in a retrieval system, or transmitted in any form or by any means, electronic, mechanical, photocopying, recording or otherwise, without either the prior permission of the publishers or a licence permitting restricted copying in the United Kingdom issued by the Copyright Licensing Agency, 90 Tottenham Court Road, London, WIT 4LP. Permissions may be sought directly from M&K Publishing, phone: 01768 773030, fax: 01768 781099 or email: publishing@mkupdate.co.uk

Any person who does any unauthorised act in relation to this publication may be liable to criminal prosecution and civil claims for damages.

British Library Cataloguing in Publication Data

A catalogue record for this book is available from the British Library

Notice

Clinical practice and medical knowledge constantly evolve. Standard safety precautions must be followed, but, as knowledge is broadened by research, changes in practice, treatment and drug therapy may become necessary or appropriate. Readers must check the most current product information provided by the manufacturer of each drug to be administered and verify the dosages and correct administration, as well as contraindications. It is the responsibility of the practitioner, utilising the experience and knowledge of the patient, to determine dosages and the best treatment for each individual patient. Any brands mentioned in this book are as examples only and are not endorsed by the publisher. Neither the publisher nor the authors assume any liability for any injury and/or damage to persons or property arising from this publication.

Coventry University Library

To contact M&K Publishing write to:

M&K Update Ltd · The Old Bakery · St. John's Street

Keswick · Cumbria CA12 5AS

Tel: 01768 773030 · Fax: 01768 781099

publishing@mkupdate.co.uk

www.mkupdate.co.uk

Designed and typeset by Mary Blood

Printed in England by H&H Reeds, Penrith

Contents

To my six-year-old son, John, who helps me to keep life in perspective

'Mummy, what are you writing about?'

'About children who find it hard to breathe.'

'How many sentences do you have to write?'

'Ummm. Quite a lot. About seven thousand I guess.'

'Seven thousand! That will take you ages. At school we sometimes do about five or six, and then draw a picture to show the rest of the story. Couldn't you do that?'

Chapter 1

Why is this book needed?

An increasing number of children and young people require long-term respiratory support. They include children who require oxygen administration, Continuous Positive Airways Pressure (CPAP), Bilevel Positive Airways Pressure (BiPAP), and mechanical ventilation. Some children need respiratory support but no other interventions or additional care, whilst others need a range of additional inputs, such as assisted feeding, specialist communication aids, and frequent drug administration. However, they all need some form of long-term respiratory support, which is primarily provided in their home.

What are the advantages of home care?

Sometimes children who require long-term respiratory support need equipment that looks as if it belonged in a hospital, perhaps even an intensive care unit, rather than in someone's home. In the past, this would usually have been the case, and these children would effectively have lived in hospitals all the time (Kirk et al. 2005). However, things have gradually changed, and the aim now is to reduce to an absolute minimum the time that children, including those who need long-term respiratory support, have to spend in hospital. The expectation is that, in the majority of cases, children's day-to-day needs, including respiratory assistance, will be provided in their homes.

Trying to avoid children being admitted to hospital unnecessarily has been on the British policy agenda since the Platt Report (1959). However, it took some time for this policy to be implemented, despite mounting evidence, such as the Court Report (Commission of Child Health Services 1976) and the Audit Commission Report (1993), indicating that children should only be cared for in hospital when this achieves something that cannot be achieved at home.

More recently, there has been a greater emphasis on children being cared for at home whenever possible, and the desirability of keeping them at home is highlighted in the National

Service Framework for Children, Young People and Maternity Services (Department of Health 2004a). This recommendation is based on a belief that children's emotional, psychological, developmental, educational and social needs are generally better met at home than in hospital, and that separation from their families (particularly their parents or primary care givers) is undesirable. These principles apply just as much to children who need long-term respiratory support as they do to other children (Balling and McCubbin 2001, Neufeld et al. 2001). In fact it is perhaps even more important for them to be supported at home because of the length of time that they would otherwise be hospitalised for. There is also some evidence that children with long-term respiratory problems enjoy better health when they are cared for at home rather than in hospital (Appierto et al. 2002).

Children who required long-term assisted ventilation were traditionally housed in intensive care units, but these are not ideal places for them to live. Such units are primarily designed for acute, life-sustaining treatment, and children who are aware of their surroundings are likely to be exposed to sights, sounds and disturbances which are not developmentally or emotionally beneficial. Both their daytime routines and their sleep patterns will probably be disturbed by noise and lighting related to the care needs of other children in the unit. There will be very little space, few play facilities, and nowhere to store toys, books or other activities. They will lack social contact because the other children will not normally be able to play or interact. Their ability to access education is likely to be limited and, at best, they will probably learn in isolation from their peers. When a child is in an intensive care unit, it is almost impossible for their parents to maintain the same type of contact and relationship with them as they would have in the family home. If a child is resident in such a unit in the long term, their relationships with siblings, grandparents and other members of their family are likely to change a great deal.

An acute hospital ward is also a less than ideal place for a child to grow up. Although the other children in acute wards are usually more responsive than those in intensive care units, they are generally acutely ill, only in hospital briefly, and not in a position to form ongoing peer relationships. Children who are hospitalised long term are also unlikely to have the same range of experiences or interactions with adults as they would encounter at home. There is very limited privacy in hospital for parents trying to establish or maintain a close relationship with their children. Whilst some parents are often resident with their child in hospital, the facilities for them are limited, and designed with short- rather than long-term stays in mind.

When a child is hospitalised long term, parents often spend a great deal of time travelling to and from hospital, and juggling the care of their child in hospital with the rest of their lives. This presents many challenges. For example, if they have other children, their relationships with the child in hospital and those at home are both likely to be disrupted. The contact between the hospitalised child and their siblings and other family members will also be limited in both time and nature. There are usually restrictions on visiting in hospitals, which can make it difficult for the whole family to be together. In addition, when their child is in hospital, parents are subject to the rules and regulations of the hospital, which can make establishing family norms problematic. In contrast, if the child is cared for at home, healthcare staff are the visitors and have an obligation to respect the family's rules, values and norms (Farasat and Hewitt-Taylor 2007).

This combination of physical, social, emotional and educational advantages makes it seem sensible for children who require long-term respiratory support to be cared for at home if at all possible. However, the advantages for the child and family are not the only reason for home care becoming the established 'norm'. There has also been an increase in the number of children who are dependent on some form of medical technology. It would no longer be feasible for all the children who require long-term respiratory support to be cared for in hospital, particularly on paediatric intensive care units. In addition, providing hospital-based care for children with this type of need, when home care is a practical option, has been described as an inappropriate use of financial resources and acute care facilities (Boosfeld and O'Toole 2000, Appierto et al. 2002). Noyes et al. (2006) nonetheless show that, whilst home care is usually the cheaper option, this is not always the case, especially if a child needs a high level of staffing but their care can be provided outside an intensive care unit. In general, however, it seems that the ideal will usually be for children who need long-term respiratory support to be cared for at home, rather than in hospital.

What are the challenges of home care?

Although caring for children at home rather than in hospital is generally seen as the best option, it is rarely an easy option for families or service providers. The challenges for parents and families whose children require long-term respiratory support are discussed in more detail in Chapters 6 to 8. Having a child who requires this type of support tends to demand a higher than usual level of responsibility and work from their parents (Parker et al. 2006, Hewitt-Taylor 2007). They often have to learn very specialist skills related to their child's requirements, develop confidence in these, and deal with the emotional workload of meeting their child's needs (Boosfeld and O'Toole 2000, Department of Health 2004b).

Having a child who needs long-term respiratory support changes their parents' lives. They may need to reorganise (and in some cases have adaptations made to) their homes, or move house, alter their employment, change their social arrangements or their arrangements for their other children, and rethink their leisure and vacation arrangements. It is often essential for parents to have assistance to meet their child's care needs, and this means that families have regular visitors to their homes, whose presence, being necessary, must be accommodated.

Whilst providing home care for children who need long-term respiratory support may be the most cost-effective option for the National Health Service (NHS), it can create a significant financial burden for the families concerned (O'Brien and Wegner 2002). Bringing up a child who requires long-term healthcare is often much more expensive than bringing up a child who does not (O'Brien and Wegner 2002, Department of Health 2004b, Parker et al. 2006). Although funding for equipment, staffing and supplies may be provided by the NHS and Social Services, parents whose children have additional health needs usually incur many expenses that they would not otherwise have. At the same time they are likely to experience financially disadvantageous changes in their employment status and decreased earning capacity (Department of Health 2004b, Hewitt-Taylor 2007).

When decisions are made as to where a child who needs long-term respiratory support will live, and how their care will be provided, the needs of the whole family should be taken into account. This includes not only the needs of the child in question, but also those of their parents and siblings, and how these will impact on one another (Hewitt-Taylor 2007). Whilst the general principle is that children are best cared for in their homes, when a child has needs which require ongoing, demanding care, and significant adaptation of family life, it may not be something that their family can manage (Carnevale et al. 2006, Parker et al. 2006). Although the child's well-being is paramount in all decisions concerning them (Department of Health 2004c), every child's well-being (including that of siblings, and how parents' well-being will impact on all their children's well-being) must be considered. For some families, caring for a child who requires long-term respiratory support in the family home is not the best option. When this difficult decision is reached, it should be respected, and families should be offered support to help them to live with it, and to continue to have meaningful and rewarding input into their child's life (Parker et al. 2006).

The wider context

This book discusses many of the day-to-day needs of children who require long-term respiratory support. This includes their physical requirements, but also their emotional, social and educational needs, and the needs of their families. The medical and technical aspects of these children's care can seem overwhelming. However, arguably the more complex and challenging parts of their management concern things that are not directly related to their physical care, such as facilitating their social needs and education. This book aims to discuss all the aspects of care that such children and their families may need, and also to place these in the context of seeing the child as a whole person and as a part of society. To achieve this, six case studies of children who need long-term respiratory support are used throughout the book.

Chapter 2 introduces these case studies and places each child at the centre when discussing the support they receive, and the ways in which their childhood and adolescence may be affected by their respiratory needs. The next three chapters discuss the physical aspects of children's respiratory needs, in terms of the problems that may create a need for respiratory support, how respiratory support may be provided, and ways in which a child's respiratory status can be assessed. Chapters 6 to 11 look at the principles of working in the home setting, working with parents, seeing the child as a part of the family, the specific needs of young people who require long-term respiratory support, working with people who are experiencing grief and loss, and some of the ethical issues involved in supporting children and young people who require long-term respiratory support.

Chapter 2

Getting to know children who require long-term respiratory support

Children who require long-term respiratory support deserve to have the same opportunities as other children (Department of Health 2004b, Whitehurst 2006). This includes being able to communicate, play, enjoy leisure and social activities, and participate in education. To illustrate these points, and also to show how different aspects of a child's needs are likely to impact on one another, the stories of six children and young people run throughout the book. They are: James, Fateha, Tom, Amelie, Aisha and Patryc.

James, who is three years old, loves more or less anything to do with trains and, as a second best, anything with wheels attached. He enjoys having baths and playing with his squirty Thomas the Tank Engine toys. He likes being read stories, especially ones about his favourite engines. He goes to playgroup once a week.

James was born at 25 weeks' gestation, and has chronic lung disease of prematurity. Because of this he needs oxygen, which he receives via nasal prongs, most of the day and at night. He also has cerebral palsy and epilepsy. His speech is a little delayed but he can speak and be understood, if people take the time to listen to him. James can walk a couple of steps using a frame, but otherwise he shuffles on the floor, uses a wheelchair, or is carried. He struggles to eat and drink enough. When he was a baby he had severe gastro-oesophageal reflux, but this has improved over time. He was fed via a nasogastric tube but has managed without this since he was two. James lives with his mother, and his five-year-old sister Alice. His father has left the family home, but Alice stays with him every alternate weekend. He visits James, but does not feel able to care for him on his own.

Fateha is now ten. When she was six, she was involved in a road traffic accident in which she sustained a fracture of her spine, which became displaced, resulting in a complete spinal cord injury at level C3. Fateha's father was killed in the accident. Fateha lives with her 12-year-old brother and her mother, who were not involved in the accident. Fateha cannot make any respiratory effort, and requires assisted ventilation, which is delivered via a tracheostomy. She is unable to move except for some very slight shoulder and head movement. She can speak, but this is difficult for her because of her tracheostomy and ventilator: she mostly communicates using a head pointer and communication aid, although her mother and one of her carers can lip-read if she mouths what she wants to say. Fateha can swallow, but has difficulty in doing so. Although she can have drinks and food if she wishes, her basic nutrition is provided via a gastrostomy.

Before her injury, Fateha enjoyed sport, dancing and singing, and was learning to play the piano. She was very popular at school. She has not returned to her previous school because the family moved house in order to accommodate the equipment and staff that she needs. She attends a mainstream school, and has a carer with her all the time because of her ventilation needs.

Tom, who is 16, likes watching sport, especially soccer, loves music, is very sociable, and enjoys spending time with his mates. He attends a local college where he is studying for his A levels.

Tom has Duchenne Muscular Dystrophy. His condition has worsened over the past few years and he is now confined to a wheelchair and requires Bilevel Positive Airways Pressure (BiPAP) at night. He has developed scoliosis and is awaiting surgery for this. He now finds it hard to play his electric guitar and his drums, because of posture and muscle weakness, and finds singing exhausting. Tom lives with his parents and his younger sister, Katie, who is 15. His older brother, Adam, also had Duchenne Muscular Dystrophy and died last year, aged 19.

Amelie, who is seven, is a high achiever at school, likes doing gymnastics and wants to start trampolining. She goes to Brownies, and has a lot of friends. Amelie has congenital central hypoventilation syndrome and requires non-invasive ventilation via a mask when she is asleep. Amelie lives with her mother, father and sister Juliette, who is ten.

Aisha, who is two, enjoys spending time with her five-year-old brother Kyle and her sister Sarah who is seven. Her favourite television programme is In the Night Garden. She loves having stories read to her, and especially likes pop-up books, and anything that makes an unexpected noise.

Aisha has Spinal Muscular Atrophy (SMA) Type I and cannot crawl, walk or sit on her own. She needs additional oxygen (which is provided via nasal prongs) during the day and has recently begun to have Continuous Positive Airways Pressure (CPAP) at night. She requires frequent suction because it is difficult for her to manage her secretions, and is fed via a nasogastric tube because she has very poor swallowing ability and a tendency to aspirate her feeds. She and her siblings live with their mother, and their father does not have any contact with them.

Patryc, who is five, loves playing with Lego, and anything to do with construction, including digging in the garden and sandpit with his toy excavators. He likes playing with water, and wants a large, pump-action water pistol for his birthday. Patryc has severe tracheomalacia, and has a tracheostomy. He lives with his mother and father.

When you work with a child who requires long-term respiratory support, apart from dealing with their respiratory needs, an important aspect of your work is enabling them to be involved in activities that they enjoy. And if you want to know what a child likes doing, you have to be able to communicate with them.

Communication

Children, including those who need long-term respiratory support, have the right to be able to communicate, not just verbally but: '…either orally, in writing, or in print, in the form of art, or through any other media of the child's choice' (Office of the United Nations High Commissioner for Human Rights 1989). Part of your role in supporting children is to find ways in which this right can be upheld. The communication that you should aim to facilitate includes verbal and non-verbal elements, and it involves how the child can communicate with you, as well as how you communicate with them.

Verbal communication includes not just the words that are spoken, but the tone, pitch, emphasis and volume of speech. Some children who need respiratory support are unable to speak. For example, although various means of helping Fateha to speak have been attempted, these have not worked for her and she uses other ways of 'talking'. Only two people can lip-read what she mouths, so she mostly uses a head pointer and a screen. Whilst this means she can state words and use icons to give extra meaning to her words, she cannot use emphasis or expression as easily as she once could. It is also more difficult for her to speak fluently because she has to either select words or icons from a menu or type them, which takes time. This makes quick responses and off-the-cuff remarks, which she was a master of before her accident, difficult. She appreciates people who give her time to make these comments anyway, or who wait for her to speak even when it takes a little longer.

She can hear well, but she cannot move unaided and finds turning her head difficult because of her injury and the ventilator attached to her tracheostomy. This means that, if people are talking nearby, she cannot look around to see who is involved in the conversation. She also finds that people often talk to her very slowly or at a level that is not appropriate for her age. She finds it very frustrating to have thoughts, feelings and questions that she cannot express, and when people speak to her as if she were much younger than she is.

Non-verbal communication includes the use of sight, gestures, movement, posture, position, touch, facial expression and eye contact. Fateha can use facial gestures and eye contact and can see well, but she cannot use other gestures because of her extremely limited mobility. To use eye contact and to see people's facial expressions and gestures, she relies on them being at her level and facing her. People often talk over her, sometimes ignoring her and only speaking to whoever is accompanying her. Because she cannot move independently, she relies on others to help her to be in the right place, and to respect her personal space. She finds that a lot of people come very close to her to speak, as if her hearing were impaired, or pat her knee or shoulder when saying hello or goodbye in a way that she finds annoying: '…as if I was a pet.'

Children who need long-term respiratory support may find it much harder to learn to communicate than other children do, and those who develop the need for long-term respiratory support may have to learn how to communicate in a completely new way. Fateha was a very fluent, spontaneous and entertaining speaker prior to her accident; she has had to learn a new, and often slow and limited way of communicating, which she does not enjoy. James finds it more difficult to articulate his words than his peers do because of his cerebral palsy. Patryc has had to learn to use a speaking valve on his tracheostomy, and it is often harder for other people to understand what he is saying than it would be with another child of his age. His mother remembers how:

> 'When Patryc was learning to talk, you could tell he knew what he wanted to say, and then after all the effort he made, people often couldn't understand him. Even now, rather than really trying to understand him, people often just say "Yes, really?" or laugh kindly or something, and that is very frustrating for him. Worst of all, some people just stop listening halfway through what he wants to say and say "Oh yes" as if he'd finished speaking.'

Children and young people who require long-term respiratory support may not have the opportunity to communicate with as many people as their peers – for example, if there are few who understand or are prepared to make the effort to understand them. Fateha has been at her current school for two years and, although her teachers are very good at working to include her, very few of them know how her communication aid works: they tend to reply on Fateha's carers for this. A handful of the children in the school know how the communication aid works, but most of them just want to see how it works as an electronic gadget, rather than to use it to listen to Fateha. There are probably only four children Fateha can have a conversation with, without her carer being involved.

If a child's mobility is restricted, it can reduce the number of people they have the chance to communicate with, and the spontaneity of their interactions. Fateha relies either on people coming to her to talk, or someone moving her to a place where she can talk to others. Because she relies on her communication aid, she also depends on others noticing cues that she wants to initiate or participate in a conversation, because she cannot interrupt or interject vocally. She spends a lot of time on the peripheries of conversations between people she would rather not be with, whilst other interactions, which she would like to be a part of, go on without her.

A variety of systems may be used to assist children to communicate, including the child lip-reading, others lip-reading the child's words, using Braille, sign language, Makaton, speech aids of various types, and thumb and eye pointing. Box 1 (below) shows links to some resources related to communication that may be useful to you and the families you work with. Whatever method is used to help a child to communicate, the degree of importance that others place on facilitating their communication is crucial. One of the greatest barriers to these children communicating is people feeling that they do not have enough time to communicate with them, or believing that this is not a priority.

Box 1: Sources of information and advice on communication

Afasic England: support for children who have speech and language difficulties, and their parents
http://www.afasicengland.org.uk/

British Sign Language
http://www.britishsignlanguage.com/

I CAN: helping children with communication difficulties to achieve their potential
http://www.ican.org.uk/

The Makaton Charity
http://www.makaton.org/

Royal National Institute for the Blind: Braille information
http://www.rnib.org.uk/livingwithsightloss/readingwriting/braille/Pages/braille.aspx

Speech Teach UK: a website providing speech therapy resources for parents and professionals
http://www.speechteach.co.uk/

Speech, Language and Communication Framework (SLCF) developed by the Communication Trust: provides practical information on communication
http://www.communicationhelppoint.org.uk/

Play

Play is a natural and essential part of every child's life. As well as being fun, play helps children learn about themselves, other people and their world; they also develop a range of emotional, motor, cognitive, social and verbal skills by playing (Skar 2002, Mulligan 2003, Sturgess 2003, Sussenberger 2003, Pierce and Marshall 2004). All children, including those who need long-term respiratory support, have the right to engage in play and recreational activities that are appropriate to their age (Office of the United Nations High Commissioner for Human Rights 1989). Some children may need more assistance than others to enable them to enjoy this right, but it is nonetheless an essential part of their lives.

Some of the challenges that have to be overcome to enable children to play relate to their mobility being restricted, either as a direct result of their physical problems or because of the equipment or interventions they need. For instance, Aisha cannot walk or crawl, so she cannot explore her environment and seek out the play activities that she wants, and she does not have the strength to pick toys up, move them, or experiment with them. Instead she relies on other people bringing her toys, and in many cases playing with them on her behalf, and showing her what they do. James loves trains but, because he needs to be attached to his oxygen supply and has mobility problems, he cannot simply set his wooden train set up on the floor. His mother has to collect the track and trains, help him to sit in a way that makes setting the track up possible, and then help him to shuffle around and set the track up and push the trains along. This does not stop him setting up and playing with his trains, but the activity requires a lot more thought, time and effort from his mother and him than it would for another three-year-old, and he cannot be left to play alone because he needs constant assistance.

A child who cannot move freely will often find it more difficult to play with the children and activities that they want to than another child would. James goes to playgroup once a week and he relies on his mother helping him get to the place he wants to be in, and with the children he wants to play with. His speech is not easy for the other children to understand, and he cannot reach out to get the toys he wants. This means that he has to ask for them, and his requests often come via his mother rather than him communicating directly with his peers. As well as affecting his play, this means that it is harder for him to learn the rules of sharing than it is for other children, because his negotiations include an adult. He also does not have the chance to develop independent relationships with other children through play in the way that his peers do (Skar 2002). His mother describes how: 'I have to try really hard to remember to get James to ask for things himself, and to ask the other children to listen to him, not me, and to try to get him talking directly to them, not via me.'

The way in which environments are designed can also affect children's ability to play. Many pieces of playground equipment are not accessible for children with mobility problems or those who need to have equipment with them, which reduces their opportunities to play, and can make them feel excluded (Skar 2002, Hewitt-Taylor 2007). Even when a child's respiratory needs do not affect their activities per se, concerns over possible problems associated with their needs can. For example, Patryc likes playing with Lego but some of the staff at his school worry about him using anything except the large bricks in case the small parts 'get into' his tracheostomy. Patryc has great and intricate construction plans, which require the smaller Lego, and he goes to great efforts to secure this. The staff also worry about him using the sandpit and getting involved in water play, particularly the children's popular activity of spraying water from the drinking fountain at each other. Patryc enjoys this a great deal, and takes every opportunity to participate.

Play activities need to be appropriate to the child's interests and cognitive level, as well as to their physical abilities, but this may require some thought and imagination: Aisha's cognitive ability is within the usual range for her age, but her very limited mobility means that making activities interesting for her requires extra thought. She enjoys being read to, and likes DVDs, although she can get bored with these. She likes toys that have different textures and that make noises and do surprising things, but someone needs to be with her to help her reach out and enjoy them, and to make sure she is well positioned to see them.

Fateha used to like sport, dancing and music, but is now unable to move. She is very limited in her play options, but computer games which she can play using her head pointer, books which she can read on screen and turn the pages using her pointer, audio books and DVDs are useful. However, it can also be very frustrating for a child who was once very physically active and sociable to have such a limited range of activities. It is also important not to make any assumptions about what children will enjoy. In the early days of her rehabilitation, Fateha was shown some DVDs of dancing, because it was assumed that she would enjoy this. She did not. It upset her to be reminded of what she could no longer do.

Social opportunities and leisure activities

Children who need respiratory support are likely to want to do the same kind of things that other children of their age do, and to engage in leisure pursuits that interest them (Department of Health 2004b, Watson et al. 2006). The difference is that they may need support, assistance and consideration by others to enable them to participate in the type of everyday activities that their peers take for granted (Watson *et al.* 2006). Disabled children are less likely than their peers to be able to meet friends outside school (OFSTED 2010), and if they cannot communicate verbally their social lives are likely to be even more limited (Watson *et al.* 2006). Fateha's mother comments:

> 'Her not being able to talk is a big thing. When you look at her, everyone thinks that the ventilator, and all her physical needs, must be hard to manage. But for a girl who used to be everyone's friend, not being able to call people over, and have a laugh, to see the people she would like to be with chatting and not be able to join in, is hard. She used to be doing something with her friends, or at some school activity or other, every evening, and now, she only has "friends" if you can call them that, at school. She never goes out with friends, or has anyone come here.'

A practical challenge for children and their families is that having a disabled child often reduces a family's income, and the cost of meeting their child's needs is generally higher than it is for other parents (Department of Health 2004b). This may mean that families have less money to spend on leisure activities. At the same time, it often costs more for children who require respiratory support to engage in leisure activities than it does for other children. They may be unable to access a full range of facilities, and suitable transport to the venues they enjoy visiting may be limited and costly (Department of Health 2004b). James loves trains, and the best days of his life are when his mother takes him out to ride on steam trains. Other local children often ride on the miniature steam railway in a nearby park, but this does not have seats that James could sit on and cannot accommodate his oxygen. He therefore has to travel just over 48 km to go on a large steam train that has full-size carriages and wheelchair access. These outings usually cost at least £60 for travel, parking, tickets for James, his mother and Alice, and incidental expenses such as drinks and snacks, compared to £1.50 per ride per person on the railway in the local park. Other children who live nearby ride on the railway in the park fairly frequently, but James usually only visits the steam trains once every eight to ten weeks because of the cost of going, and because it entails a full and exhausting day out.

As well as increasing the cost of leisure activities, and the frequency with which they can engage in these, a lack of accessible facilities in their neighbourhood can mean that children who require long-term respiratory support do not have the chance to socialise with their local peer group in the same way as other children (Department of Health 2004a). The practicalities of a child's needs can also alter their ability to socialise with their peers. Tom's friends from college like to spend Saturday evenings on the local recreation ground, and although Tom cannot do some of the things they do, such as skateboarding and cycling, he enjoys being with them. His friends are usually happy to collect him, or his mother will take him there, but he also relies on someone being able to wheel him around on the rec and then take him home, or on his mother or one of his night carers coming to collect him. Parents are not a part of the ethos of the recreation ground gatherings. Now that he requires BiPAP at night, he feels less able to stay out late because his carer starts work at half-past nine. This makes it even harder to ask one of his mates to take him home, and break up their evening. One of his carers will come and collect him, but this is a goodwill arrangement, not something she has to do. He can also decide to start his BiPAP late, but that means that his carers are at home doing nothing until he arrives, and invites comments from his parents.

Sometimes a child's additional respiratory needs create unexpected difficulties in relation to their social lives. Amelie loves gymnastics and her school recently organised a trip to London to see a display. Amelie wanted to go. However, as it was over 100 km away, there was some concern that she might fall asleep in the minibus and need assisted ventilation. She could only go if her mother was able to accompany her as a helper, and she had to have her ventilator with her. There was also the question of having enough space in the minibus for the ventilator. This was achievable, but it meant that Amelie could not assume, as her peers did, that she could go. Amelie was once regularly invited to sleepovers but it soon became common knowledge that she could not go to them. Group sleepovers seem impossible: Amelie cannot sleep with a group, because she needs her ventilator and carer. She can have one friend at her house for a sleepover, but she still needs her ventilation set up at night and a carer there, and it might be difficult for her friend to sleep with all this going on. She cannot go to friends' houses because she would need her ventilator and a carer or her mother to accompany her, and few of her friends' houses could accommodate this. The main purpose of a sleepover is for the children involved to have a relatively erratic overnight sleep, without much adult supervision, and this is not really an option for Amelie.

Education

All children have a right to education, and their education should include more than just the quest for academic achievement (Russell 2003). It should be directed towards '...development of the child's personality, talents, mental and physical abilities to their fullest potential' (Office of the United Nations High Commissioner for Human Rights 1989).

Children who require long-term respiratory support have the same right to education as other children, and they should have an equal breadth of educational experience (Berry and

Dawkins 2004). If a child or young person cannot attend school or college, this may affect not just their academic achievements but also their chances to socialise with their peers. Their presence in mainstream education also gives their peers an opportunity to accept them as people, value them, learn to see them as a part of society, and to develop an ethos of inclusion (Berry and Dawkins 2004). In the UK the intention is that, wherever possible, children should be enabled to learn in a mainstream education environment, unless the child's parents or guardians decide against this, or it is incompatible with the efficient education of other children, and no reasonable steps can be taken to prevent that incompatibility (OFSTED 2004).

The Disability Discrimination Act (HMSO 2005) requires schools not to treat disabled pupils less favourably than others and to make 'reasonable adjustments' to ensure that they are not disadvantaged. It is nonetheless important to stress that children with additional needs must be given the support they need, in order to make mainstream education meaningful for them and genuinely inclusive (Russell 2003, Berry and Dawkins 2004). If a child cannot participate in most activities that other pupils are engaged in, they are not really included. Indeed, this may even detract from an inclusive ethos and cause them to be seen as different, or segregated (Hewitt-Taylor 2007).

Achieving the ideal of inclusion can be challenging, because there may be some things that children who need respiratory support cannot do. Fateha attends a mainstream school, but most of her communication is channelled via her carer because few of the pupils or teachers know how to use her communication device. She cannot participate in sports, although she would love to, because she is immobile. When she joined the school, there were discussions about what Fateha would do during physical education sessions. Initially the suggestion was that she could watch, but she did not enjoy this: it reminded her of what she could not do, and she did not find watching the other children very interesting. Her mother now tries to co-ordinate any appointments she needs with PE sessions, although this is not always possible. When she is at school for PE, she and her carer do other activities together, such as going for a walk in the school grounds.

Fateha cannot eat lunch with her peers because, although she sometimes has small drinks or tastes of food, she is mostly fed using a gastrostomy. There was debate as to whether she would sit in the cafeteria to have her gastrostomy feed alongside the other children, so that she was included in lunchtime activities, but Fateha prefers to have her feed away from the other pupils. Whilst being with them might increase her inclusion in their lunchtime, she felt that she would rather not have others watching and commenting on her feeds. These two issues illustrate how there may be no single answer to some aspects of inclusion. The decisions made were the ones that were right for Fateha, to make her feel as comfortable as possible in the school environment.

Although there are significant limits to Fateha's inclusion because of what she cannot physically do, she can join in with some activities with her peers. She does the same academic work as them. Although it can take her longer to complete her work (because she has to use her head pointer), she achieves very well. She finds it hard to be really involved in any discussions because of her lack of verbal options, but does have the input from other pupils to consider in her own work. When the class does group or pair work, she is always included in a group or pair, and in these situations she is able to participate more fully. On balance, she and her mother decided that, whilst she would never be able to fully participate in all her peers' activities, she would still be best placed in a mainstream school where, with her carer, she could participate in some activities with her peers.

Sometimes it is necessary to acknowledge that schools cannot completely include children in every activity, but the aim is to maximise inclusion and to make education as meaningful as possible for each individual child. Amelie's class expects to be going on a two-day residential outdoors activities event when she is in year four. Amelie wants to go, and, although this will mean arranging for her overnight ventilation needs to be met, the school are doing their best to make it happen. However, there will still be some limitations on what she can be involved in. The plan is that Amelie's mother will stay with her at night, because the location is outside the geographical area that her carers can work in. Amelie will not be able to sleep in the dormitory with the other children because her mother and the ventilator cannot be accommodated there. Usually, she is no different from her peers, and although she wants to go she is already worried that she will be left out because she will have no part in the night-time fun in the dormitories, which her friends will spend most of the day discussing. Plans for this trip, and anxieties about it, are already underway for Amelie, although it is still more than a year away. Her mother is very clear that:

> 'Ultimately it will be Amelie's choice. If she decides that not being there at night is going to make her feel so left out during the day that she will be unhappy, then she doesn't have to go. She wants to go so she can be a part of it, and if she feels she will be less a part of it being there but restricted than by not being there, she doesn't have to go. At the moment we are all busy making sure she is included, but we have to make sure that it's what she wants, not an agenda to include her at all costs.'

Sometimes children who need respiratory assistance have a number of absences from school because of ill-health. However, they may also miss many hours of school because of the health-related appointments they need to attend (Department of Health 2004b, OFSTED 2010). Enabling children to participate fully in education includes keeping their absences to a minimum by effective planning of appointments, but this can be difficult to achieve. Fateha's mother tries to get appointments for times when she is timetabled for activities that she cannot participate in, but this does not always fit the available appointment times.

Children and young people may need specialist transport to get to school or college, either because of the type of transport they need or how far they live from a suitable school or college. The availability of transport can therefore affect their education, and can particularly impact on their extracurricular activities (Berry and Dawkins 2004). Children with additional needs should be enabled to participate in all the activities the school offers their peer group, including extracurricular activities (HMSO 2005). However, even when a school seeks to meet the requirements of the Disability Discrimination Act (HMSO 2005), a lack of suitable transport or staffing issues can create difficulties. For instance, Fateha discovered that there was a school chess club, and was interested in joining as she can use a computer program to play chess, and can use her communication aid to ask her carer to move the pieces on a real chessboard. The teacher who runs the chess club was happy to help set things up so that she could attend, but Fateha's transport could not be arranged at different times, and her support staff change shifts around school time schedules, so she has been unable to join in.

For a child's education experience to be as good as possible, there needs to be collaboration and co-operation between health, social care and education services, aimed at meeting the child's needs and aspirations (OFSTED 2010). You may find yourself well placed to act as a link between services, and to help them work together to achieve the outcomes that are important to the child or young person you work with.

Privacy

The United Nations Convention on the Rights of the Child (Article 16) states that 'No child shall be subjected to arbitrary or unlawful interference with his or her privacy, family, home or correspondence...' (Office of the United Nations High Commissioner for Human Rights 1989). Privacy includes physical privacy, privacy of thoughts, feelings and emotions, and privacy in communication with others. Children who require respiratory support have the same rights as other children, and the staff who work with them have an obligation to respect their privacy. However, they may still find achieving privacy very difficult. For example, Fateha requires a carer or other adult to be with her all the time, and every response she makes, every feeling she expresses, every gesture or activity, can be observed by another person. Amelie's 'private space', her room, is, of necessity, seen and intruded upon on a regular basis by her carers. She sometimes feels that her choices (for example, of posters, toys, and clothes) are commented on by people whose opinions she does not want.

The nature of the care that some children or young people need may require disclosure of personal details of their life and private facts about their body (Olsen *et al.* 2005). Tom is finding the physical care he requires more intrusive as he gets less able, and as he gets older. He now uses BiPAP at night, and it has taken him some time to get used to having a carer within hearing distance when he is asleep. His friends sometimes take girlfriends home after an evening out, but this does not seem a possibility for him, with his carer awaiting his return and wanting to start his BiPAP.

A child or young person who requires respiratory support may therefore have limitations on their privacy, in comparison to their peers. Supporting them effectively includes considering ways in which these limitations can be reduced to the absolute minimum, and exercising sensitivity and respect in handling private information and intimate knowledge of them and their lives.

Summary

The assistance you provide for children and young people who need long-term respiratory support should focus on meeting their needs as children or young people, and as members of a family, not just their medical or technical needs. This involves finding out what their preferences are, and maximising their opportunities to do things that they enjoy. It means learning to communicate with them, making the effort to do so, and encouraging others to do so. It is also important to create opportunities for children to engage in play activities and leisure pursuits, and to spend time with any peers they may want to socialise with. Part of your role may also be helping children and families to access the right education provision for them, planning their support in a way that will help them to achieve what matters to them, and working with them on achieving the maximum possible level of inclusion. You should also be aware of the limitations that children's needs may place on their privacy, and seek to reduce your intrusion on them and their families to the minimum level possible.

Chapter 3

Why children need long-term respiratory support

The body needs a way of getting oxygen and getting rid of carbon dioxide. Breathing does both these jobs, which is why we all have to breathe, or to be attached to some form of technology that will do the job for us, in order to survive.

We need oxygen because, along with carbohydrates, it creates the energy that our bodies need in order to function. The process of oxygen and carbohydrate producing energy can be expressed by the chemical equation:

$$C_6HI_2O_6 + 6O_2 = 6CO_2 + 6H_2O + Energy$$

Carbohydrate plus oxygen makes carbon dioxide and energy

This equation shows that oxygen and carbohydrates act together to release the energy that is vital for the body's processes, and also that the combination of carbohydrates and oxygen does not only produce energy. Carbon dioxide is also formed in the process, and if there is too much carbon dioxide in the body it becomes harmful. So, if a person's breathing is not effective, the body will not receive enough oxygen to meet its energy needs, and will not get rid of enough carbon dioxide. The results of this will depend on the severity of the breathing problem. Things may work a little less efficiently if it is a minor problem. However, if breathing ceases altogether, the person will die within minutes because the vital organs (such as the heart and brain) have no energy with which to work.

Fateha cannot breathe at all: if her ventilator failed, and another method of providing her with oxygen was not established, she would die within minutes. Tom, on the other hand, can breathe reasonably well during the day. Over time his respiratory muscles tire and, especially at night, his breathing is not efficient enough to take in enough oxygen and dispose of enough carbon dioxide. Because of this, he uses BiPAP to assist him to breathe adequately at night. He began using BiPAP because his breathing was getting worse, but if he did not have BiPAP for one night it is unlikely that he would die because of it. His body would accumulate higher levels of carbon dioxide than it should, and have lower levels of oxygen than it needs, and he would feel unwell. However, at this point in time his BiPAP is not critical to his immediate survival in the same way as Fateha's assisted ventilation.

Breathing occurs via the respiratory tract, or airway. The airway is often described in two parts: the upper and lower airway (see Figure 1 (below) and Figure 2 (page 24)).

The upper airway

The section of the airway from the nose and mouth to the end of the larynx is usually called the upper airway; and the section from the trachea to the end of the bronchioles is referred to as the lower airway.

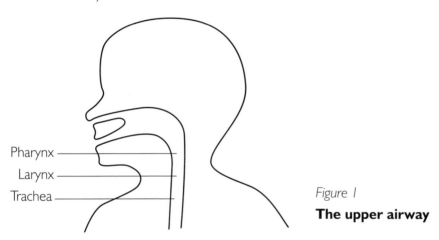

Pharynx
Larynx
Trachea

Figure 1
The upper airway

Air enters our bodies via our noses and mouths. Babies who are less than six months old can only really breathe through their noses, so if a small baby gets a blocked nose they may not be able to breathe because they have no other options. As the air enters the nose and mouth, it starts being warmed by body heat. It is also moistened, and filtered by the tiny hairs (cilia) that line the airway. This process continues throughout its journey to the lungs.

After the nose and mouth, the air arrives at the pharynx. The upper part of the pharynx is where the Eustachian tubes from the ears emerge, and where the tonsils live (Saladin and Miller 2004). The Eustachian tubes are much straighter in young children than they are in adults, so it is much easier for infections to spread between the upper airway and the ears.

The mouth and pharynx accommodate food and drink as well as air, and the airway does not become separated from the gastrointestinal tract until just before the next part of it: the larynx. The epiglottis, which sits slightly above the larynx, covers the airway during swallowing as a means of preventing food and drink from entering the lungs. Movements of folds of cartilage at the top of the larynx also prevent food or drink from entering the airway (Saladin and Miller 2004). There are situations in which the risk of children's food or drink entering their lungs (aspiration) is increased. James had severe gastrointestinal reflux, where some of the contents of his stomach regurgitated into his upper gastrointestinal tract, with a risk that they would travel far enough upwards to enter the airway (Allen 2010). Aisha has Spinal Muscular Atrophy (SMA), a neuromuscular disorder, in which the impulses or instructions sent from the brain via motor nerves (nerves that carry messages from the brain to the muscles) are either not transmitted, or not transmitted fully. There are over 20 motor nerves in the brainstem (an area at the base of the brain) and they have to fire their messages in sequence for a normal swallow to occur (Allen 2010). Because these impulses may not all arrive successfully at their target muscles when a child has SMA, it is not surprising that Aisha finds swallowing difficult.

Aisha is now fed using a nasogastric tube, partly because of her swallowing problems. However, this can create its own difficulties. A nasogastric tube is inserted through the nose and its tip rests in the stomach, so feeds are delivered directly to the stomach. However, because the tube at first passes through the nose and pharynx, there is a risk that, rather than passing into the oesophagus and stomach, it will instead pass into the larynx and onwards into the lungs. This is one reason why the position of a nasogastric tube always needs to be checked after insertion and before use: to make sure that the tube is in the stomach, not the lungs.

The larynx houses the vocal cords. We usually speak by passing air over our vocal cords as we breathe out, so damage to the larynx can affect a child's voice. Laryngitis means 'inflammation of the larynx' and this is why laryngitis affects the voice. However, the larynx is not the only part of the airway responsible for sounds. The pharynx, mouth, lips and tongue all refine the sounds produced by the vocal cords (Saladin and Miller 2004).

The lower airway

The trachea follows on from the larynx, and is supported by 16–20 C-shaped rings of cartilage (Saladin and Miller 2004). The open part of the C faces towards the child's back, and means that the oesophagus, which is located behind the trachea, can expand to allow food to pass through.

Sometimes, the tissue that makes up a part of the airway is either damaged or not formed correctly. The effect of this depends on the part of the airway that is damaged, and the nature and extent of the damage. If a child has tracheomalacia, as Patryc does, some of the cartilage in the trachea is absent, small, malformed, or too pliable. This means that the affected part of the trachea is underdeveloped, constricted or floppy, and it is difficult for air to move past the damaged portion. Some children need surgery or some form of respiratory assistance to manage this problem and enable them to breathe. Patryc's tracheomalacia was so severe that a tracheostomy was needed to overcome the obstruction it caused. He now breathes via the tracheostomy, rather than through his nose and mouth.

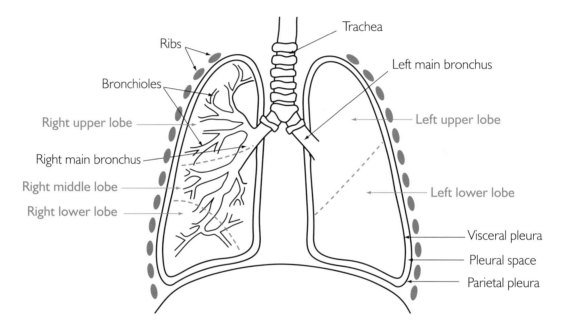

Figure 2 **The lower airway**

A tracheostomy is an incision in the trachea that enables a child to breathe or to receive assisted ventilation. A child may need a tracheostomy because they have an obstruction to their airway above or at the level of their trachea, as Patryc does. In other situations, as in Fateha's case, a tracheostomy is used as a means of providing assisted ventilation. As discussed in Chapter 5, it is not always necessary to have a tracheostomy to provide long-term assisted ventilation (Amelie uses non-invasive ventilation, which is provided via a mask rather than a tracheostomy) but some children have a tracheostomy for this purpose.

If a child breathes through a tracheostomy, the functions of the airway above this level are lost. Because the larynx is above the level of a tracheostomy, having a tracheostomy affects a child's voice because air is both taken in and passed out via the trachea, and does not pass over the vocal cords in the usual way. A tracheostomy bypasses the upper airway, and thus the humidification, moistening and filtering, which this part of the airway provides, is lost. This increases the risk of infection because micro-organisms are less likely to be filtered out, and the air that enters via a tracheostomy is drier than it would normally be at this point. Sometimes a filter system, such as a Heat Moisture Exchanger (sometimes called a 'Swedish nose' or 'thermovent') is used on a tracheostomy, to reduce these problems. Anything which inadvertently enters the airway via a tracheostomy, such as particles or irritants, has less distance to travel to reach the lung tissue than if it were inhaled through the nose or mouth. Some of the staff at Patryc's school worry about him playing in the sand or with water in case these get into his tracheostomy. This is not a reason for him not to play in the sand or with water, but it is probably sensible for them to be aware of the slightly increased risk of these particles inadvertently getting into his airway.

At the end of the trachea the airway divides into two. This point is known as the carina, hilum, or bifurcation of the trachea. The two parts into which the airway divides are called the bronchi (or the right main bronchus and left main bronchus). The right bronchus is the wider and more upright of the two (Saladin and Miller 2004). This means that it is slightly easier for anything that has inadvertently got into the child's airway to pass into the right bronchus than the left (Saladin and Miller 2004).

The right and left bronchi each divide into branches, one of which goes to each lobe of the relevant lung. (The lungs are divided into lobes, which are separated from each other; the left lung has two lobes, and the right has three.) Each branch then subdivides into smaller and smaller branches, finally becoming bronchioles. The smallest bronchioles eventually become a single layer of cells known as terminal bronchioles. The bronchioles end in alveoli, which are small, irregular-shaped sacs, where the transfer of oxygen from the environment into the bloodstream, and the removal of carbon dioxide from the bloodstream, occurs. So, although air is taken into the body through the mouth or nose, it does not really start to become usable until it reaches the alveoli. Anything that reduces the amount of air that gets this far reduces the amount of oxygen that is made available to the body. Anything that stops carbon dioxide from leaving the alveoli prevents carbon dioxide being expelled from the body.

The alveoli

The alveoli are located at the end of the bronchioles and are like miniature, irregular-shaped balloons (see Figure 3, page 26). They fill with air when we breathe in and deflate as we breathe out. However, ideally the alveoli should not deflate completely when we breathe out. If they do, then it is harder for the body to take the next breath (Sly and Collins 2006). If you think how hard it is to blow up a balloon that has no air in it at all, compared to one that has a bit of air in to start the process, you can see how useful it is for the alveoli to remain very slightly inflated between breaths.

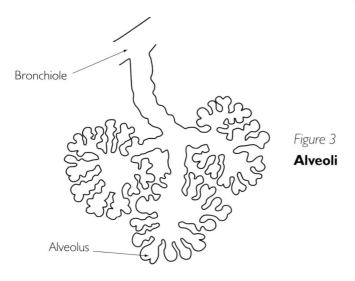

Bronchiole

Alveolus

Figure 3
Alveoli

One thing that helps prevent the alveoli from completely deflating (or collapsing) at the end of each breath is surfactant. Surfactant is a substance that is produced in the alveoli and spreads across their inner surface like a lining. Surfactant is secreted during gestation, but not until the foetus is about 30 weeks, and it does not achieve its mature state until approximately 36 weeks gestation (Smith et al. 2010). Very premature babies, such as James, are born before usable surfactant has been produced, and may therefore be given artificial surfactant when they are born.

Before babies are born, their lungs are not used for breathing. The oxygen they require is supplied via the placenta, and carbon dioxide is also removed in this way. The alveoli are not developed to their ideal functional form before about 32–36 weeks gestation (Smith et al. 2010). James was born at 25 weeks' gestation, and his alveoli had not yet developed enough for him to use them to breathe effectively, so he needed assisted ventilation. It also seems that when babies are born extremely prematurely, their alveoli do not develop as would be expected after they are born (Sweet et al. 2002). This is partly because the lungs are forced to take on a task that is not really appropriate for their age, and they cannot develop as they should whilst they are doing this extra work. It is also partly because, as described in Chapter 5, providing assisted ventilation often puts greater pressure on lung tissue than normal breathing does. James needed assisted ventilation for several weeks after he was born and this caused some unavoidable damage to his alveoli. If he had not received assisted ventilation, he would not have survived, so there was no other option. Assisted ventilation techniques have in fact improved greatly. However, as babies survive earlier and earlier premature birth, it becomes harder to supply assisted ventilation without any damage being caused to their alveoli.

Premature babies like James often need to be given additional oxygen as well as receiving assisted ventilation. Although we all need to take in enough oxygen, getting too much of it can damage body tissue. The body has natural antioxidant systems to protect it from being damaged by excess oxygen, but these are not fully developed in premature babies (Philip 2009). Premature babies may therefore also sustain alveolar damage from receiving high oxygen concentrations.

A lack of natural surfactant, having to use their alveoli for gas exchange, needing additional oxygen, and receiving assisted ventilation can all therefore combine to cause injury to premature babies' lung tissue. The inflammatory effects of such injury may also result in long-term damage to lung tissue. When babies are born extremely prematurely, as James was, this combination of factors can contribute to what is sometimes termed 'chronic lung disease of prematurity': lung disease that occurs because of their premature birth, and that continues to affect them in the long term.

Airway muscles

The width of the respiratory passages can be altered by contraction or relaxation of the muscles in their walls. Muscle constriction narrows the airways, whilst relaxation increases the available width. This affects the volume of air that can reach the alveoli because, if the airways are narrowed, less air can get in. The smallest parts of the airways (the smaller bronchioles or alveoli) do not have any muscle tissue. But the airways that do contain muscle tissue are above the alveoli, so muscle contraction still affects how much air gets into the alveoli, and how much air can escape. Muscle contraction can be very useful for preventing irritants from progressing through the airways, but in some situations it can become problematic. For example, the symptoms of asthma are caused by inflammation of the airways and excessive constriction of the muscles of the bronchi and larger bronchioles (bronchoconstriction). This means that when a person has an asthma attack, the airways are narrowed by both inflamed airway tissue and constricted muscle tissue, and less air can get in and out. The wheezing heard in asthma is the sound of air trying to move through a constricted airway. Salbutamol, a drug commonly used to treat asthma, counters the airway muscle contraction and dilates the bronchi (which is why it is called a bronchodilator), thus allowing more air to get in and out of the lungs.

Oxygen and carbon dioxide exchange

For oxygen to get into the body and for carbon dioxide to leave, air needs to arrive in and leave the alveoli. However, getting air to and from the alveoli does not guarantee that the body's tissues receive oxygen and get rid of carbon dioxide. Every part of the body needs oxygen, and for this to happen the oxygen needs to move from the alveoli into the bloodstream and be carried around the body. Similarly, carbon dioxide needs to be collected from every part of the body and transported in the blood back to the alveoli for disposal.

Every alveolus is surrounded by a network of tiny blood vessels (capillaries), which collect oxygen for delivery to the body and drop off carbon dioxide for removal. If anything interferes with the blood supply around the alveoli, even if a child is breathing in a good amount, their body may not get enough oxygen, because it cannot get into the bloodstream. Similarly, they may not be able to get rid of enough carbon dioxide.

The air that we breathe in is made up of more or less whatever is in the atmosphere. The gases in the air we breathe in are approximately:

- Oxygen: 21%
- Carbon dioxide: 0.04%
- Nitrogen: 78%
- Inert gases: 0.96%
- Water vapour: varies

Although the air from the atmosphere is what we breathe in, by the time it reaches the alveoli it is more humidified and has also mixed a little with carbon dioxide on the way, so the percentage of oxygen in the alveoli is actually quite a bit less than the 21% in the atmosphere. However, the air that arrives in the alveoli has a high oxygen and low carbon dioxide concentration, compared to the concentration of gases in the blood that is returned from the body to the alveoli. Gases tend to diffuse from an area of high concentration to an area of low concentration. Oxygen therefore tends to diffuse into the blood vessels around the alveoli, which have a much lower oxygen level, and carbon dioxide tends to diffuse from the alveolar capillaries into the alveoli, where the carbon dioxide level is lower (see Figure 4 below).

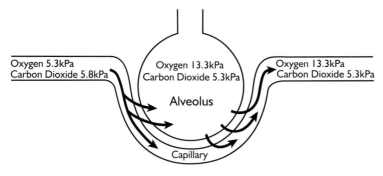

Oxygen 5.3kPa
Carbon Dioxide 5.8kPa

Oxygen 13.3kPa
Carbon Dioxide 5.3kPa

Oxygen 13.3kPa
Carbon Dioxide 5.3kPa

Alveolus

Capillary

Figure 4 **Gas exchange**

In healthy children, the alveolar membranes, which oxygen and carbon dioxide have to cross, are very thin and easy for the gases to diffuse through. However, if anything makes these membranes thicker or harder to get through, such as the scarring from repeated infection (which Aisha has) or the damage from prematurity (which James has), it is harder for oxygen and carbon dioxide to diffuse. If a child has a lot of secretions in their alveoli, then it is harder for oxygen and carbon dioxide to move because they have to get through the secretions as well as the alveolar and capillary walls (see Figure 5 below). Aisha and James both get repeated chest infections, and the secretions from these make it harder for carbon dioxide to be removed efficiently from the body and for oxygen to be taken up as easily as usual.

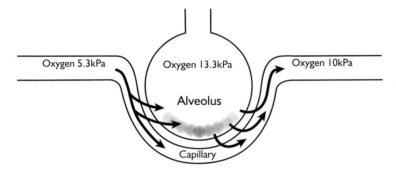

Figure 5 **Gas exchange where secretions are present**

The amount of oxygen and carbon dioxide in the blood is not usually expressed as a percentage but as a partial pressure. Partial pressure means the part of the total pressure of all the gases present that a particular gas represents. The partial pressure of oxygen therefore refers to the part of the total pressure of gases represented by oxygen. Normal atmospheric pressure is 760 mmHg or 101.3 kPa. That means that the partial pressure of oxygen in the air at normal altitude, at 21% of 101.3 kPa, is 21.173 kPa. If atmospheric pressure falls, the partial pressure of gases will fall (because the total pressure is smaller, each part will also be smaller), although their percentage will not. This is why it is harder to breathe at high altitude.

Sometimes you will hear a child's blood gases being discussed. This refers to the partial pressure of gases in the blood. The right numbers for these depend on where the blood is taken from. If the blood is from an artery, then the numbers should resemble those that you would find in the alveolar air during inspiration. As stated above, the oxygen level in the alveoli is quite a bit lower than in atmospheric air, and the usual partial pressure of arterial oxygen is about 10–14 kPa (Lynes and Kelly 2009). If the reading is taken from venous blood, it will be lower in oxygen because the veins transport blood that is relatively low in oxygen and high in carbon dioxide back to the lungs. If the carbon dioxide level in the blood is higher than normal, it suggests that either the body is creating more carbon dioxide than usual, or that the carbon dioxide is not being excreted effectively from the lungs. If the oxygen level is lower than normal, it suggests that oxygen is either not being delivered effectively to the alveoli or not being taken up effectively by the alveolar capillaries.

Haemoglobin

Blood is made up of red blood cells, white blood cells, platelets and plasma. The partial pressure of gases described in a blood gas reading refers to the gases dissolved in the plasma. However, although carbon dioxide is mostly carried in the plasma and some oxygen is also carried this way, most of the body's oxygen is carried by red blood cells (haemoglobin). Haemoglobin that is carrying oxygen is called oxyhaemoglobin. This means that, for the body to get enough oxygen, sufficient oxygen has to enter the body, there has to be a method of getting it from the alveoli to the blood vessels around the alveoli, and there need to be enough red blood cells to carry the oxygen around the body.

The pleura

The alveoli, bronchioles and bronchi are the functional parts of the lungs. They are supported by connective tissue, and enclosed in, and separated from, the rest of the body by a sac called the pleura (see Figure 2, page 24). The pleura is made of two layers, with a small amount of serous fluid between them. The inner layer (the visceral pleura) attaches to lung tissue, and the outer layer (the parietal pleura) adheres to the inside of the chest wall, including the ribs and the upper surface of the diaphragm. The fluid between the layers is just sufficient to prevent friction but not to interfere with lung function. Usually there is no space between the pleural layers, and they function together to provide friction-free movement of the lungs when we breathe. However, if air gets into the space between the pleural layers (a condition known as a pneumothorax), it separates the two layers, the suction pull that prevents the lung tissue collapsing (see page 31) is lost, and some of the lung tissue then collapses. Any collapse of lung tissue means that air cannot enter or leave the lungs efficiently, so the body's supply of oxygen is reduced and the removal of carbon dioxide is lessened. The effect a pneumothorax has on a child depends on its size and location.

Another problem that can occur within the pleura is a pleural effusion, where the pleural space has a build-up of fluid rather than air, which again decreases the suction pull, and compresses lung tissue. Children may also develop infection or inflammation in the pleura (pleurisy), which creates friction during the usually friction-free movement of the pleural layers while breathing. This may impair a child's breathing – because the inflamed pleura makes their breathing less effective and because the pain of the friction means that they cannot breathe freely.

Breathing

For oxygen to enter the body and carbon dioxide to leave, air has to move in and out of the respiratory passages. This is achieved by movement of the respiratory muscles. The main respiratory muscles are the diaphragm and the intercostal muscles. The diaphragm is located at the base of the ribs and the intercostal muscles are located between the ribs (see Figure 6 below). They attach to the parietal pleura, which surrounds the lungs. These muscles contract and then relax and, because they are attached to the pleura, the lung tissue moves with them.

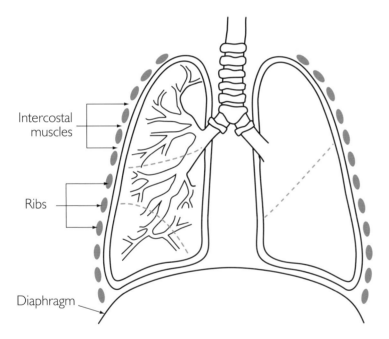

Intercostal muscles

Ribs

Diaphragm

Figure 6 **The respiratory muscles**

The first rib is fixed in place, and when the intercostal muscles (the muscles between the ribs) contract, the other ribs are pulled up towards the first one. This means that they move upwards and outwards. When the diaphragm muscle contracts, the diaphragm moves downwards (Singh 2005). As the diaphragm and ribs are attached to the parietal pleura, this moves with them. The movement of the parietal pleura creates a negative pressure or suction pull within the pleura, so the visceral pleura follows its movement. This suction pull is then applied to the lung tissue, effectively stretching the hollow airways upwards, downwards and outwards, and making them wider (Nicolai 2006). The alveolar walls are stretched, and there is more space in the alveoli. There is now space available in the airway. This means that the pressure within the lungs falls below the pressure in the atmosphere, because there is the same amount of air in them, but more space for it to spread out. To try to make the pressures equal again, air moves from the atmosphere into the airways without any conscious effort on our part (except now, when you are reading about it!). So, air moves into our lungs to fill a space, rather than being forced into them, as it is with a balloon. When children receive assisted ventilation the process is different, as described in Chapter 5.

When the time is right, the respiratory muscles relax, and the ribs, diaphragm and lung tissue returns to their previous position. This means that there is less space in the airways, and air naturally flows out. Then it all starts again. Figure 7 (below) illustrates the movement of the ribs and diaphragm during inspiration and expiration. This cyclical process is described as the respiratory cycle: inspiration (breathing in and getting more oxygen), followed by expiration (breathing out and getting rid of carbon dioxide).

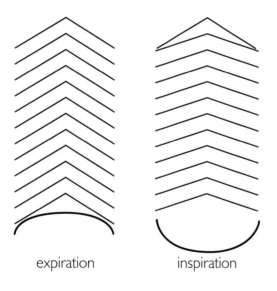

expiration   inspiration

Figure 7

Movement of ribs and diaphragm in breathing

In healthy adults, who are not doing anything particularly strenuous at the time, this happens about 14 times a minute. In babies it happens up to 50 or so times per minute (MacGregor 2008). Babies' metabolic demands, and thus their need for oxygen, are higher in relation to their body size than those of adults. At the same time, their lungs are much smaller and move less efficiently so they have to breathe more often. Their ribs and diaphragm muscle fibres insert more horizontally than adults' do, which means that they have proportionally less movement and therefore less increase in lung volume for each muscle movement (Nicolai 2006). Their diaphragms are flatter than adults', so they get less change in volume each time their diaphragm contracts than an adult does (Nicolai 2006).

Figure 8 shows the difference in the amount of volume gained by a respiratory movement in an adult compared to one in a small child. Babies also have a much more pliable chest wall than adults, so their lungs are not held expanded as strongly as adults' are (Sly and Collins 2006). This all means that they have to breathe more frequently, and work harder to do this, than healthy adults. Life is not fair for children.

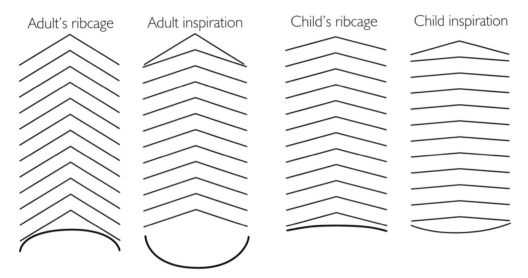

Figure 8 **Comparison of adult and child inspiration**

Because the movement of lung tissue relies on muscle movement, muscle problems can affect breathing. Aisha has SMA, which means that the messages that should be sent to her respiratory muscles by her motor nerves (to request that they contract) are not conveyed effectively, and the muscles do not contract as well as they should. In SMA, the intercostal muscles are particularly affected, so Aisha relies heavily on her diaphragm for breathing. However, any alteration in posture that affects the movement of the ribs or diaphragm can also affect breathing. Aisha finds it hard to sit upright, because SMA also affects the muscles that enable her to do this. This means that, in addition to the messages instructing her respiratory muscles to move being diminished, her ribs and diaphragm will not be well positioned for movement. For every muscle movement she makes, her lungs are therefore likely to expand less than one would expect. Tom's scoliosis alters the position of his ribs, so the movement of his intercostal muscles will not necessarily cause the same change in lung volume as it otherwise might, and his position can place pressure on his diaphragm and make its movement less efficient. So, any muscular or neuromuscular disorder, or postural problem, which affects the ribs or diaphragm, can affect a person's breathing.

It is possible to consciously breathe air in, to try to bypass obstruction, but it is more difficult to force air out past an obstruction. This means that when a child has some obstruction of the airway, however hard they work to breathe in, they may not be able to expel air effectively. So, even if they can force air into their airways, air with a high oxygen content cannot reach the alveoli because the 'old air', which they cannot force out, remains there. It also means that carbon dioxide stays in the body.

Lung compliance

For the lungs to expand and air to get in, the intercostal muscles and diaphragm have to move; but for the width of the airways to increase, so that air moves into the lungs, the airway tissue also needs to be able to stretch. The stretchiness of lung tissue is referred to as 'lung compliance'. If lung tissue is less stretchy than you would expect, then the lungs are described as 'stiff' or having 'decreased compliance'. Scarring of the lung tissue, for example in James's case from when he was a premature baby, or in Aisha's case from repeated chest infections and feed aspiration, may cause decreased compliance.

Reduced compliance makes breathing harder because, if the airways do not stretch very well, the muscle movement causes less of a change in space inside them, and less air enters at each breath. However, perhaps even more problematic than getting air in is that (rather like damaged elastic) non-compliant lung tissue does not spring back very well. Making extra muscle movement may enable a child to create enough pull to stretch their lung tissue, even if it is harder work. However, although you can work hard and stretch something that is not very stretchy, it is much harder to make it bounce back. James may be able to take forced breaths to stretch or expand his alveoli, but forcing them to contract is harder. If air is forced into the body but cannot then be forced out, air is trapped in the respiratory passages, and cannot leave. This means that air with a high carbon dioxide level does not leave the lungs as well as it should, and that there is less room, when the lungs expand again, for new, oxygen-rich, air to get in. It also means that secretions, which usually move with the elastic recoil of lung tissue, do not move as well, which makes the child more prone to chest infections.

Control of respiration

We know how air gets to the alveoli, and what needs to move to make that happen. However, that still leaves the question of how we know when to breathe. Usually, we do not decide to breathe. It just happens. It is also impossible for most of us to decide to stop breathing and to carry this on for very long. Breathing is controlled by a number of things and is not a completely conscious choice, although you can consciously tweak it, as you are probably doing now – because you are reading about it.

We mostly know whether or not to breathe because of the levels of carbon dioxide and, to a lesser extent, oxygen, in our blood. In healthy people the main stimulus for breathing is rising carbon dioxide levels in the blood. However, in some long-term conditions, where carbon dioxide levels are constantly high, falling oxygen levels can become the main stimulus.

The monitoring of oxygen and carbon dioxide levels in the blood is carried out by chemoreceptors (receptors that deal with chemical information and which are sensitive to carbon dioxide and oxygen levels in the blood). However, these receptors cannot act on levels of oxygen and carbon dioxide directly. They have to pass this information on to the brain, which has to receive this information, organise it and pass instructions to the relevant muscles for a breath to be taken. Stretch receptors in the bronchi, bronchioles and visceral pleura also monitor the inflation of the lungs and relay this information to the brain for action (Saladin and Miller 2004). Irritants in the airway can stimulate the vagus nerve, which passes this information to the brain and initiates the impulses associated with coughing and constriction of the bronchi (Saladin and Miler 2004). So breathing is affected by a number of stimuli and monitoring systems, but co-ordinated by the brain.

Areas in the part of the brain called the brainstem (the pons and medulla) are described as controlling breathing. However, several other areas of the brain also contribute to breathing control. These include the limbic system and the hypothalamus, which are involved in pain and emotion affecting breathing – for example, anxiety may trigger hyperventilation (Saladin and Miller 2004). Any significant damage to the brain, and especially any damage which has an impact on the brainstem, can therefore impair or even stop breathing.

If the evidence from all the relevant sources suggests that a breath is needed, the brain sends an order (or nerve impulse) to the respiratory muscles to request this. To get from the brain to the intercostal muscles and diaphragm, these messages have to travel via the spinal cord. This means that an injury to the spinal cord can affect breathing because the messages get as far as the spinal cord but do not reach the intercostal muscles or diaphragm. The impulses that pass the messages to the diaphragm to request movement are the third cervical nerves (C3). Those that pass the request to the intercostal muscles are the fourth, fifth, sixth and seventh thoracic nerves (T 4–7). Because Fateha has a spinal injury at C3, any messages that are sent to this level and below are not passed on, so the messages from her brain requesting a breath are not sent to her diaphragm or intercostal muscles. This means that she cannot breathe because there is no way of the message from her brain to her respiratory muscles being transmitted. If her injury were lower, for example at level C5, then the messages would be sent to her diaphragm but not her intercostal muscles, so she would have some respiratory muscle movement but might still need respiratory assistance of some kind.

If Fateha had sustained this injury directly from the accident she was involved in, she would probably have died, because her breathing would have stopped immediately. However, although she sustained a fracture to her spine during the accident, her spinal cord was not initially damaged. The complexity of removing her from the vehicle resulted in the fracture becoming displaced and injuring her spinal cord. At this point, there were paramedics available to provide assisted ventilation, so she survived, but cannot now breathe on her own.

Although breathing happens automatically, we can deliberately affect our breathing, for example by taking a deep breath. This voluntary control of breathing is organised by a part of the frontal lobe of the brain, and bypasses the respiratory centre in the brainstem in order to send messages (impulses) directly to respiratory neurones in the spinal cord (Saladin and Miller 2004). Voluntary control does have its limits. It cannot do the whole job of breathing: it does not work when we are asleep or not in a position to remind ourselves to breathe, and we cannot hold our breath until we die. There is a breaking point at which automatic control takes over (Saladin and Miller 2004).

Amelie has congenital central hypoventilation syndrome (CCHS). This is a genetic condition in which the control of breathing has some disordered function. Exactly what goes wrong with breathing control in CCHS, and why this happens, is not completely known (Weese-Mayer et al. 2010). It seems to be a complex disorder in which the respiratory control mechanisms in the brainstem do not respond in the expected way to the information provided by chemoreceptors about the levels of oxygen and carbon dioxide in the blood. In a 'typical' situation, when a child with CCHS is awake, other influences (such as the voluntary control mechanism that bypasses the brainstem and respiratory stimulants such as the limbic system) seem to compensate for this. Although the child takes shallower breaths than usual, their breathing is adequate. However, when they go to sleep and these influences are diminished, their breathing stops.

The extent to which children are affected depends on the severity of the disorder. Some children can never breathe unaided; others breathe well when they are awake but only take very shallow breaths when they are asleep. The most commonly quoted picture is Amelie's: she breathes when she is awake, but stops breathing when she falls asleep. This is why she needs assisted ventilation when she is asleep but not when she is awake. CCHS may appear to improve or become more manageable as the child gets older, but the condition does not actually improve

(Weese-Mayer *et al.* 2010). Other respiratory control mechanisms become more developed as a child gets older, and the situation becomes more manageable as they sleep less, or with a more predictable pattern, but the underlying disorder remains unchanged.

Tissue oxygenation

Finally, if everything goes to plan in the lungs and there is enough haemoglobin to carry the oxygen and a strong enough heartbeat to pump the blood round the body, oxygen-rich blood arrives at the tissues, and oxygen can be dropped off and carbon dioxide picked up. Gas exchange in the tissues occurs between the capillaries and the fluid surrounding the tissues. Gases again diffuse from high concentration to low concentration so that oxygen from the capillaries diffuses into the tissue fluid and then enters the cells. Carbon dioxide from the cells moves into tissue fluid and then diffuses into the capillaries (see Figure 9 below). The haemoglobin that is carrying oxygen (oxyhaemoglobin) breaks up relatively easily to release oxygen to the cells. The blood, which now contains a high level of carbon dioxide and less oxygen, returns to the alveoli, and the carbon dioxide diffuses into the alveoli and is excreted.

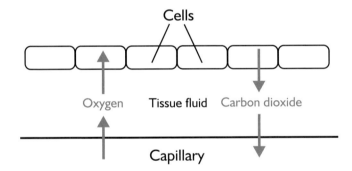

Figure 9 **Tissue oxygenation**

Do children grow out of breathing problems?

When children have, or develop, respiratory problems, people often discuss whether or not they will 'grow out of it'. Sometimes they do, but more often the problem remains but becomes less important as the child grows and other things compensate for it. As we grow, our airways become wider and their tissues become stronger, so they collapse less readily. This may mean that problems such as tracheomalacia, which Patryc has, appear to improve. The basic defect in the tracheal cartilage usually still exists, but the symptoms and consequences become less severe because there is proportionally more tracheal cartilage that has developed after the injury and which supports the damaged part. As a child grows, their tracheal cartilage becomes stronger, and thus the undamaged cartilage can better compensate for, or support, the damaged element.

Like everything else, children's airways get bigger as they grow, so anything that blocks the airway can become less significant, as long as the blockage does not get bigger with it. If a child has a 1 mm blockage in an airway which is only 5 mm wide that is pretty serious. However, if they have a 1 mm blockage in an airway that is 10 mm wide it is slightly less troublesome, all other things being equal. The number and size of bronchioles and alveoli also increase with age so the child has more compensatory capacity because, even if the same number of alveoli or bronchi remain damaged, there are more undamaged ones to compensate. Children's metabolic rate, and therefore oxygen consumption, falls as they get older, so they are not living 'on the edge' so much, in terms of needing to breathe fast to keep up with their metabolic demands. The chest wall becomes stronger and harder as a child grows, and they develop more accessory muscles so they can better compensate for respiratory compromise. As the ribs and diaphragm take on their adult structure, each breath moves the lungs more efficiently, so the work of breathing is reduced. Children therefore often appear to grow out of respiratory problems, or their problems seem to improve as they get older, even if their physiological problem actually remains unchanged.

However, in some cases respiratory problems worsen as a child gets older. As they grow, the child's increasing weight, and the size of their chest, creates a greater workload for the respiratory muscles. Any muscle weakness or deterioration in muscle strength may therefore be additionally challenged by a heavier workload. Problems such as scoliosis may worsen as the child gets older, and any impact that this has on their chest movement may therefore increase. Tom's scoliosis is worsening, and this, combined with his muscles getting weaker at the same time as his body size and weight are increasing, means that his chest expansion is gradually reducing.

Repeated chest infections may cause increasing lung damage and children who find it hard to clear their secretions may develop chronic infection. In such children, not only is alveolar tissue scarred, but there is also an almost permanent volume of debris and secretions through which oxygen and carbon dioxide have to attempt to diffuse. A child like Aisha, who has a degenerative neuromuscular disorder, will find that their condition worsens as they get older. Aisha will have progressively less functional motor neurones (the nerves that pass instructions about muscle movement from the brain to the relevant body part) as she gets older, and her condition, and therefore her breathing, will get worse, not better. Thus, whilst some children need less respiratory support as they get older, others need more.

When you are supporting children and their families, it is important to see them as people, not conditions to be treated or managed. However, it is also important to know why they have the physical needs they do, and how their health condition affects them. It may be useful for you, or the children and families you work with, to access resources specific to the health condition their child has. Some examples of these, which are relevant to the children discussed in this book, are shown in Box 2 below.

Box 2: Organisations that offer information and support related to specific conditions

Aid for Children with Tracheostomies
http://www.actfortrachykids.com/

BLISS: a charity offering information and advice for parents of premature babies
http://www.bliss.org.uk/

Breathe On UK: a national charity dedicated to supporting the families and carers of young people who require long-term ventilation
http://www.breatheon.org.uk/

British Lung Foundation: information on children's lung diseases
http://www.lunguk.org/you-and-your-lungs/childrens_lung_disease/

Congenital Central Hypoventilation Syndrome (CCHS) Support Group
Email: cchssupp@hotmail.com

Head Injury Association
http://www.headway.org.uk/home.aspx

Muscular Dystrophy Campaign
http://www.muscular-dystrophy.org/

SCOPE: a national disability charity that focuses on people with cerebral palsy
http://www.scope.org.uk

Spinal Injuries Association
http://www.spinal.co.uk/

Spinal Muscular Atrophy: Families of SMA
http://www.fsma.org/

Spinal Muscular Atrophy: The Jennifer Trust for Spinal Muscular Atrophy

http://www.jtsma.org.uk/

UK Children on Long Term Ventilation

http://www.longtermventilation.nhs.uk/

Chapter 4

Ways of providing respiratory support

The assistance that children may need with their breathing varies. It may include them requiring: additional oxygen, Continuous Positive Airways Pressure (CPAP), Bilevel Positive Airways Pressure (BiPAP), and mechanical ventilation. This chapter describes these different types of respiratory support, why they may be needed, and how they may help individual children.

Oxygen administration

Usually the oxygen in the atmosphere is enough to meet the body's needs, but sometimes children need more than this, and are given additional oxygen. Children may need extra oxygen for a number of reasons. Aisha has had problems with repeated aspiration of feeds, and has frequent chest infections, both of which are likely to have caused damage to her lung tissue. James has damage to his lung tissue caused by prematurity. So, even when enough oxygen reaches James and Aisha's alveoli, it does not diffuse into the capillaries as easily as it would if their lung tissue was not damaged. If the percentage of oxygen that they breathe in (and therefore the part of the total pressure of gases which it exerts on the alveolar walls) is a bit higher than it would usually be, the difference between the partial pressures of oxygen in the alveoli and the capillaries surrounding the alveoli is higher. It is therefore more likely that oxygen will pass through the alveolar walls (see Figure 10 on page 42. This is why both James and Amelie are helped by having extra oxygen.

It is also harder for oxygen and carbon dioxide to move across the alveolar walls if the child has a lot of secretions in their alveoli, because the gases have to get through the secretions as well as the alveolar and capillary walls. This is why children may need oxygen when they have a chest infection, but not at other times, or may need more supplementary oxygen at some times than others. Whilst Aisha and James always need some extra oxygen, when they have an acute chest infection they need more additional oxygen than usual.

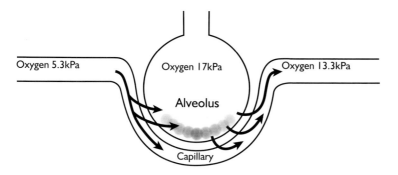

Oxygen 5.3kPa

Oxygen 17kPa

Oxygen 13.3kPa

Alveolus

Capillary

Figure 10 **Gas exchange where secretions and lung tissue damage are present**

A child can receive additional oxygen via either a mask or nasal prongs. If oxygen is required in the long term, it is usually given via nasal prongs, especially if it is being given to an infant or small child at a flow rate of 2 litres per minute or less (Balfour-Lynn *et al.* 2009). Nasal prongs are flexible tubes that deliver oxygen into the child's nose. They are usually much easier to keep in the right position than an oxygen mask, especially on babies or small children, and are less cumbersome. This is how both James and Aisha receive the extra oxygen they need. Low flow nasal prongs can actually deliver up to about 4 litres per minute of oxygen, but babies and small children can rarely tolerate more than 2 litres per minute, because a higher flow is not comfortable (Balfour-Lynn *et al.* 2005). The oxygen from the nasal prongs and the oxygen from the air that the child breathes in through their mouth mix, so although nasal prongs will deliver a certain amount of oxygen, the concentration that the child takes in also depends on how much they are breathing through their mouth (McGloin 2008).

When children need oxygen long term, at home, it is usually provided by using an oxygen concentrator rather than oxygen cylinders. This is what James and Aisha use. An oxygen concentrator takes in ambient air, absorbs the nitrogen from it (which increases the percentage of oxygen in the remaining mixture of gases) and then delivers the concentrated gases, which are high in oxygen, to the child (Lynes and Kelly 2009). This means that the oxygen that is produced is used up immediately, not stored, and there is an easily available supply from the atmosphere (Lynes and Kelly 2009).

Although a concentrator is the most common way of providing oxygen in the home, if a child requires a very high concentration of oxygen they may need cylinders or other methods of supplying it (Balfour-Lynn *et al.* 2009). In addition, oxygen concentrators are not usually suitable for use outside the home, and it is always advisable to have a back-up supply in case of the concentrator malfunctioning, so even when children use oxygen concentrators, they also need to have a portable and back-up oxygen supply available (Balfour-Lynn *et al.* 2009).

Giving a child extra oxygen does not get rid of carbon dioxide, but it can help reduce the level of carbon dioxide in the body, because if the body has enough oxygen it makes less carbon dioxide. If the body is not getting enough oxygen to meet its metabolic needs, it uses what is called anaerobic metabolism: 'anaerobic' means 'without air'. This is a good solution for brief episodes when oxygen is in short supply, or when demand outstrips supply. However, it is a much less efficient process than using oxygen, and it produces a lot more waste products, including carbon dioxide and other acids. Getting enough oxygen therefore cuts down on how much carbon dioxide is produced, but does not reduce it immediately or directly.

The air we breathe is quite moist and fairly warm, depending on the temperature outside. We have probably all been out early in the morning in winter and felt the difference between breathing the relatively warm air indoors and the sudden blast of cold air from outside. Sometimes when you go to a higher altitude or a very dry environment you can feel the lack of humidity. If a child receives additional oxygen from a concentrator or cylinder, the natural humidity and warmth which air gets from the atmosphere is reduced. Oxygen itself can make the airway dry, especially if it is given in high volumes or concentrations (McGloin 2008).

Cold, dry air stops the cilia (the tiny hairs that line the airway) from working properly. The jobs of cilia include wafting any foreign material, and moving mucus, so that it does not build up and can be removed fairly easily from the respiratory tract. So, if the function of cilia is disturbed, the child has a greater chance of getting respiratory infections. This is why some oxygen delivery systems have a humidifier or warmer in them. Balfour-Lynn *et al.* (2005) suggest that when children are receiving more than 1 litre per minute of oxygen, humidification should be considered, partly for comfort as well as to reduce the risk of infection. However, children who are at home and have less than 1 litre per minute of oxygen flow (as James and Aisha do when they are well) do not always receive humidification. This is because it is thought that the oxygen mixing with the ambient air, which they breathe in through their mouths, should provide enough humidity to overcome the problem (Lynes and Kelly 2009).

Continuous Positive Airway Pressure (CPAP)

Sometimes, when a child has a problem with their breathing, additional oxygen is all they need. However, this is not always enough. If there is an obstruction of some kind in the airway, or if the muscles that make the lung tissue move are not working well enough, however much oxygen you give, it will not get to where it is meant to as efficiently as it should. CPAP can sometimes be useful in this type of situation.

CPAP means Continuous Positive Airway Pressure. It does what it says: applies a continuous pressure inside the airways. It does not give the child any breaths, but it provides a permanent, very low pressure to keep the airways open (Williams and Asquith 2000, Morton *et al.* 2005). Figure 11 (below) shows where CPAP occurs in a child's breath. If you liken the lungs to a balloon, it is like someone constantly applying just enough pressure to keep the balloon a tiny bit inflated. The pressure is applied throughout the airways, so it is useful for keeping the upper airways open if they have tendency to collapse, as well as keeping the alveoli open. If a child has mild airway obstruction, a bit of pressure applied to the inside of the airway can be enough to keep it open, overcome the obstruction and make sure that the child can use the oxygen they take in. For example, for some children who have mild tracheomalacia, CPAP provides enough pressure to overcome the obstruction or stop the 'floppy' part of the airway from collapsing when they breathe out. Unfortunately, Patryc's tracheomalacia was too severe for this to work and he required a tracheostomy to bypass the affected part of his airway.

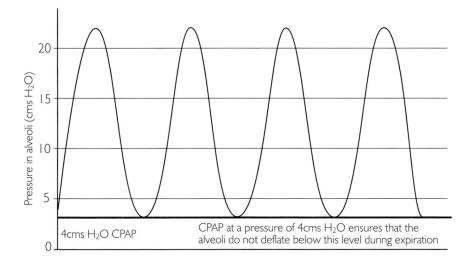

Figure 11 **Occurrence of CPAP in a child's breath**

As well as overcoming mild structural airway obstruction, CPAP makes breathing easier. The alveoli are not meant to deflate fully at the end of each breath. If they do, then the work of breathing is much greater. If a child has a tendency for their alveoli to collapse more than they should, then CPAP can be used to keep them inflated the right amount. If the child gets tired easily because their respiratory muscles are weak, CPAP can be very useful for keeping the alveoli very slightly more inflated than usual at the end of each breath. This means that the child has to make less effort and expend less energy to inflate their alveoli at each breath, which reduces the overall workload of their breathing. For Aisha, the combination of her respiratory muscles not working as well as other children's, and her postural problems meaning that some parts of her airway may be mildly obstructed, makes CPAP useful. Everyone's respiratory effort is reduced when they sleep, and for children like Aisha this can mean that their problems become more severe at night. In addition, when she is lying down, it is harder for her respiratory muscles to move her body weight. This is why she needs CPAP at night but not during the day.

The amount of CPAP a child receives is described in terms of how much pressure is provided. This is measured in centimetres of water (cm H_2O) because it describes the pressure that would be required to move a certain volume of water. CPAP usually starts at between 3 and 5cm H_2O but this can be increased if the child's condition necessitates it (Marcus et al. 2006). Although CPAP provides pressure to the airways, it does not mimic breathing; it just provides one constant pressure. For the lungs to inflate and deflate again, the child has to breathe. The carbon dioxide levels in the blood, and all the other things that tell the child to breathe, still need to make this happen. It is just that the airway and alveoli are held slightly open.

Pressure support (Trigger)

If a child has weak respiratory muscles, or the mechanisms that tell them to breathe are working, but not very effectively, they may not breathe deeply enough to inflate the alveoli very well. If the alveoli do not inflate fully, then not enough oxygen will get into them, and not enough will be delivered to the body. Pressure support can help with this because it provides extra pressure at the end of each breath to ensure that the alveoli do inflate enough (Williams and Asquith 2000, Morton et al. 2005).

Pressure support therefore gives the child assistance at the opposite end of a breath from CPAP. Figure 12 (see page 46) shows how pressure support works. CPAP stops the airway and alveoli from collapsing at the end of expiration (breathing out), and pressure support makes sure that the alveoli inflate fully when the child breathes in (inspiration). Like CPAP, for pressure support to work, the child has to take the breaths they need. It does not supply breaths; it just supplements the ones that the child takes.

Pressure support works by sensing how much pressure change there is in the child's airway (roughly, how big an in-breath they are taking). When the child has inflated their lungs a certain amount (or created a certain amount of pressure change in their lungs), the ventilator 'tops up' the breath. This is also sometimes referred to as 'trigger' because, by making a certain amount of respiratory effort, the child 'triggers' the machine to give them a top-up to make their breath big enough or deep enough. In some cases the trigger level, or amount of pressure the child has to create, is very low, and they are given almost all the breath, but the key thing is that they have to make it clear that they want to take a breath, and make some respiratory movement.

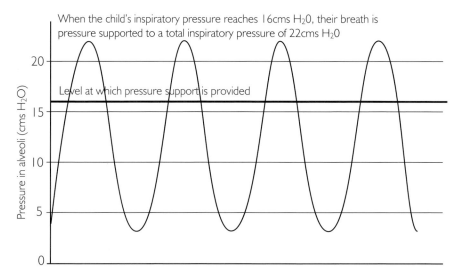

Figure 12 **How pressure support works**

The amount of pressure support provided is also described in terms of the pressure given, but in this case it is the pressure that the lungs will be inflated to, not the amount of pressure delivered by the machine alone. When you pump up your car tyre, the reading you get is the final pressure, not how much you put in, and that is how it works with pressure support. In a well child, the pressure in the lungs at the end of inspiration is usually around 22–24 cm H_2O, but this varies, depending on the state of the child's lungs.

Bilevel Positive Airways Pressure (BiPAP)

BiPAP (Bilevel Positive Airways Pressure) (Jaarsma et al. 2001) is a bit like a combination of CPAP and Pressure Support. It does the same job as CPAP, from the point of view of providing a constant pressure within the airways, so that they are held open and the alveoli are kept slightly inflated (or slightly more inflated than usual), but it also tops each breath up so that reasonably good alveolar expansion is achieved, as happens in pressure support. In BiPAP, the child initiates all their breaths; unless they give an indication that they want to breathe, nothing happens, but the workload is reduced at both 'ends' of the breath (Morton et al. 2005). Figure

13 (below) illustrates this process. Tom has recently started to use BiPAP. This works for him because he can breathe, but his muscle weakness is increasing, and it is getting harder for him to move his respiratory muscles enough to take breaths that are sufficiently deep. This is especially problematic when he is asleep; his respiratory responses are lessened because he is asleep, and his weight is less well supported when he is lying down than when he is sitting. BiPAP provides assistance with inflating his lungs, which means that he gets a better amount of air into his lungs each breath, and this and his airways being held slightly open at the end of expiration means that the workload of his breathing is reduced.

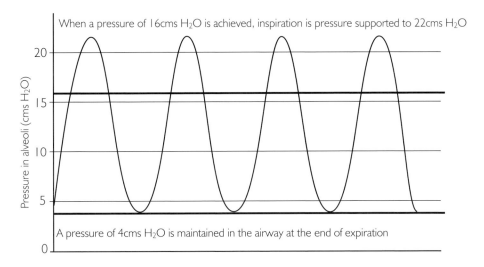

Figure 13 **Bilevel Positive Airways Pressure (BiPAP)**

The pressures given in BiPAP are, not surprisingly, a combination of the pressures seen in CPAP and pressure support. These are expressed as the inspired pressure achieved over the level of CPAP, for example: 22/4 cm H_2O.

Mechanical ventilation

Pressure support, CPAP and BiPAP can be described as 'assisted ventilation' because they all help with a child's breathing. However, they do not give the child any breaths. They just help, to varying degrees, with the work of the breathing that the child is doing. Fully assisted, or mechanical, ventilation involves giving the child some or all of the breaths they need. Fateha uses this because she cannot breathe at all. CPAP, BiPAP or pressure support would not work for her because there would be no breaths for them to act on. Usually, the type of mechanical ventilation used is called positive pressure ventilation.

Positive pressure ventilation provides the child with breaths, inflates the lungs, and delivers oxygen to the alveoli, but it does so in quite a different way from the way we usually breathe. Although the lungs are sometimes likened to a balloon inflating, they are not inflated in the same way as a balloon; the movement of the rib cage and diaphragm mean that there is more space in the airways and air is sucked in. In positive pressure ventilation, the lungs are inflated by the ventilator 'pushing' air in, so assisted ventilation more closely resembles a balloon being inflated. The ventilator delivers pressure that inflates the lungs to a certain, set, pressure. The breath then stops and air flows out of the lungs, but the ventilator maintains a set pressure at the end of each breath so that the alveoli do not deflate completely (Hewitt-Taylor 2008). This process is shown in Figure 14 (below). In this way, positive pressure ventilation uses pressures that are similar to BiPAP. The difference is that the breaths are initiated and delivered by the machine; the child receives a whole breath, not just assistance with their own breath.

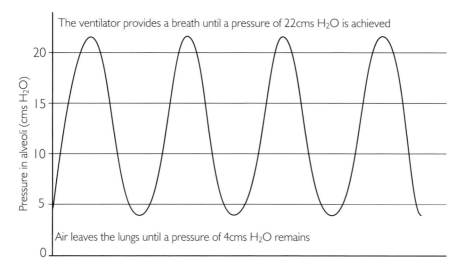

Figure 14 **Positive Pressure Ventilation**

The pressures given for positive pressure ventilation are:

- An inspired pressure (the pressure to which the lungs will be inflated). This is most commonly referred to as the peak pressure, the inspired pressure, or IPAP (Inspired Positive Airways Pressure).
- The pressure that is maintained in the lungs at the end of each breath. This may be called PEEP (Peak End Expired Pressure) or EPAP (End Positive Airways Pressure) (Hewitt-Taylor 2008).

As in BiPAP, these pressures are expressed as the inspiratory pressure over the expiratory pressure, for example 22/4 cm H_2O.

Although positive pressure ventilation provides breaths, it does not always mean that the ventilator does all the child's breathing for them. There are many different ways in which mechanical ventilation can be provided. These are often referred to as modes of ventilation.

Modes of ventilation

Sometimes children can take breaths for themselves, but cannot reliably take as many as they need, and even providing some assistance, for example by using CPAP or BiPAP, is not enough. In this situation, the ventilator may be set to deliver a proportion of the breaths the child needs, but also to allow them to take some breaths themselves. For example, if they are of an age and size to need 30 breaths a minute, but cannot manage this, the ventilator will perhaps deliver 15 and the child will be expected to take 15 or so. Usually, in this type of ventilation, the ventilator will fit in with what the child is doing, rather than the child having to try to work around the ventilator. This way of providing assisted ventilation is sometimes called Synchronised Intermittent Mandatory Ventilation (SIMV), or synchronised ventilation – because the ventilator synchronises with the child (Morton *et al.* 2005).

Sometimes in synchronised ventilation, the ventilator will definitely deliver a set number of breaths, but more often it will check how many breaths the child is taking and deliver up to its set number, depending on what the child does. For example, if the aim is for the child to get 30 breaths, and the ventilator is set to deliver 15, if the child takes 20 breaths, the ventilator will provide 10 so that the child gets 30 breaths in total. However, if the child only takes 10 breaths, the ventilator will still only provide 15. Sometimes the ventilator is set to be able to give all the breaths the child needs (for example, 30) but will synchronise with the child and deliver up to 30, depending on how much respiratory effort the child makes. This can be useful for children like Amelie because, whilst she needs the ventilator to deliver all her breaths while she is asleep, as she wakes up she begins to breathe. It is therefore useful if the ventilator can work with her as her respiratory rate changes, so that she gets enough breaths but not too many.

If a child cannot breathe at all, the ventilator will be set to give all the breaths they need (Williams and Asquith 2000). For example, Fateha cannot breathe at all, so the ventilator is set to give her all the breaths she needs. There is no point in giving her options for breathing on her own, because that is not going to happen. However, if this was done when someone could do some breathing themselves, it would make life very uncomfortable because they would effectively be 'fighting' the ventilator to try to breathe. When the ventilator delivers all the breaths, and does not allow the person to breathe at all, it is called Controlled Mandatory Ventilation (CMV) or controlled ventilation.

These are all quite nice, neat definitions of different types of ventilation. However, real life is not always nice and neat. Sometimes a mixture of pressure support CPAP, BiPAP and assisted ventilation is used. For example, some children need CPAP during the day but synchronised ventilation at night when their respiratory effort is less. Others need CPAP during the day and BiPAP at night. Some children have a combination of what sound like two different things at the same time: for example, SIMV and pressure support. This means that the child receives some 'full' breaths from the ventilator, and these breaths will synchronise with any breaths they take for themselves. In addition, any breaths that the child takes for themselves are pressure supported, or 'topped up'. For example, let's say it has been decided that the total number of breaths the child will need in a minute is 30, with 15 synchronised breaths and the rest pressure supported. If the child takes 15 breaths, these 15 will be pressure supported and the other 15 will be given by the ventilator. If they take 20, these will all be pressure supported and the ventilator will give 10 full breaths. If the child takes all 30 breaths themselves, these will all be pressure supported. This mode would be called SIMV and pressure support, or synchronised ventilation with pressure support, or something similar. There are also other variations on modes and mixes of modes, but these are the basic principles of assisted ventilation.

Mask versus tracheostomy

When CPAP, pressure support, BiPAP or mechanical ventilation are used, the pressure and mix of gases that will be delivered is created in a machine, and then has to be delivered to the child's airway. Between the pressure and mix of gases being created in the ventilator machine, and it getting into the airway, there has to be very little chance for the gases to escape. If any of the gases sent from the ventilator escape before they reach the airway, the pressure delivered will be lower than it should be, and the mix of gases may be affected. For this reason, the system that delivers the gas mix from the ventilator to the child has to be air-tight.

In acute situations, when a child is critically ill, this is usually achieved by using an endotracheal tube (ETT): a tube that is inserted through the nose or mouth and that ends just above the bifurcation of the trachea (see Figure 15 on page 51). The ETT is secured in place and the ventilator is attached to it. This is quite an effective way of making sure that the pressure sent by the ventilator reaches the lungs, but is really only suitable for fairly short-term use. If a child requires longer-term ventilation, something else is needed.

In the past, long-term assisted ventilation was usually achieved by using a tracheostomy. A tracheostomy is an artificial opening into the trachea, which allows air to enter and leave the airway. To keep the tracheostomy from closing or becoming blocked, a rigid or semi-rigid tube (known as a tracheostomy tube) is inserted into the opening and held firmly in place, using some kind of securing system, often ties or velcro. Tracheostomy tubes have been developed over the years to make them softer, more flexible, easier to maintain, and less damaging to the airway.

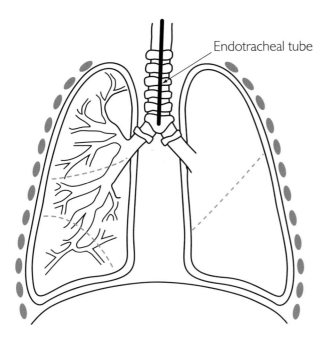

Endotracheal tube

Figure 15 **Position of a endotracheal tube**

Patryc has a tracheostomy because the extent of his tracheomalacia meant that he could not use his upper airway to breathe. However, Patryc does not need assisted ventilation, because his respiratory muscles and lung tissue are undamaged; he breathes atmospheric air through his tracheostomy and can breathe frequently and deeply enough himself. Fateha, on the other hand, receives assisted ventilation via a tracheostomy. Her ventilator attaches directly onto the tracheostomy tube and the pressure from the ventilator is transmitted into her airway by this route. She had no damage to her airway, but a tracheostomy was considered to be the best way to provide her with assisted ventilation.

Although tracheostomies can provide long-term assisted ventilation, over the past two decades there has been an increasing use of what is termed 'non-invasive ventilation'. This means ventilation that does not require an invasive procedure such as a tracheostomy. Non-invasive ventilation is delivered via a tight-fitting mask that covers the nose or nose and mouth, or via a specially designed nasal prong. The mask or prong has to be well enough secured, and has to adhere sufficiently to the contours of the face or nose so that no pressure escapes. These masks can be used for mechanical ventilation, CPAP and BiPAP.

Both methods of providing assisted ventilation (the mask and the tracheostomy) have advantages and disadvantages. Having a tracheostomy creates a permanent change in the child's appearance, whereas non-invasive ventilation means that, when the child does not need assisted ventilation, they have no distinguishing features and do not require the kind of additional consideration that having a tracheostomy can necessitate. For Amelie, who only needs assisted ventilation whilst she is asleep, using a mask means that during the day she is no different from her friends, whereas with a tracheostomy she would have a permanent stoma on her neck, and would probably need to be more cautious about a number of the activities that she enjoys.

Having a tracheostomy means that the child's breathing is carried out via the trachea, and the functions of the airway above this point are lost. It also means a reduction in humidification, less protection from infection, and that air entering the body has a shorter distance to travel and consequently any foreign objects, infective organisms or irritants have a shorter distance to travel before reaching the lungs. A tracheostomy tube may become dislodged or blocked, which means that the child's breaths may not arrive in the airway. If the tube becomes dislodged it may also cause trauma to the airway. Although someone with a tracheostomy can still cough, clearing their secretions may be more difficult, especially if they have a speaking valve or Heat Moisture Exchanger ('Swedish Nose') on the tube.

A tracheostomy also affects a child's speech. Whilst it is difficult to speak when mask ventilation is being delivered, a child who only requires ventilation at night, as Amelie does, can speak as usual during the day if they use non-invasive ventilation. If Amelie had a tracheostomy, she might be able to use a speaking valve, which is a type of tracheostomy tube valve that allows air to be inhaled into the tracheostomy but exhaled over the larynx so that the child can produce sounds (NHS Quality Improvement Scotland 2008). However, it would mean that her speech sounded different from that of her peers. With a disorder where the child's ventilation needs may reduce as they get older, it may be preferable to avoid using a tracheostomy, as no tracheostomy closure will be necessary when the child is weaned from ventilation.

However, using a mask or nasal prong to deliver assisted ventilation has its challenges. It is necessary to be able to secure the mask or prong well, and for some children who have postural problems and/or poor head control, this can be problematic. Although most ventilator masks have very pliable gel seals, there are some children whose facial anatomy or posture makes it very hard for them to achieve a good seal. If achieving a good seal is problematic, and the child is very dependent on the ventilator, then it may be impractical to use mask ventilation. It may be more effective and safer to rapidly and securely attach the ventilator to a tracheostomy.

The pressure required to deliver assisted ventilation can mean that using a mask is noisy and uncomfortable. The feeling created by the pressure has been likened to placing your head outside a car window on a motorway. When a child requires ventilation at night, it can be difficult for them to learn to sleep with this sensation. Aisha took a long time to get used to mask ventilation; and for some children the discomfort is not tolerable, and they prefer a tracheostomy. In addition, whilst a mask leaves the child free to speak as normal when they are not receiving assisted ventilation, they may find communication very difficult whilst ventilation is in progress. A tracheostomy is used to provide Fateha's ventilation because she requires this 24 hours a day and depends on it completely. She cannot speak because she cannot detach her tracheostomy from the ventilator, but if she used mask ventilation she would need to have the mask in place 24 hours a day, so she would still not be able to speak. Because she also uses a head pointer, attaching this and her mask would probably be quite cumbersome. With a tracheostomy her face is kept exposed, and although she cannot talk she can make facial expressions, and her mother can lip-read what she says, both of which would probably not be possible with a mask.

Personal preference and tolerance of different systems are very important considerations when choosing how assisted ventilation should be provided. Whilst a tracheostomy is often seen as being the more invasive option, and it is true that masks and nasal prongs have improved over time, neither option is intrinsically better; what is best is what best meets the individual child's needs and preferences.

Risks associated with assisted ventilation

There are problems associated with providing any form of positive pressure ventilation, be it CPAP, BiPAP, pressure support, or full mechanical ventilation. These problems also exist whether assisted ventilation is provided by mask or tracheostomy. A lot of the risks are due to the differences between how we usually breathe and how a ventilator works in terms of pressure.

It is very hard to inflate alveoli to just the right pressure when you are pushing air in, instead of letting it flow in to fill the available space in the lungs. It is therefore quite easy for slightly too much or too little pressure to be given. If the pressure is even slightly too high, then the alveoli are stretched more than they should be. This matters because, if they are overstretched then, like any piece of overstretched elastic, they eventually lose their elasticity. Putting too high a pressure against the alveolar walls also means that they can become damaged. Pushing hard against any body tissue damages it, and the alveoli are no exception. As with any balloon, if too much pressure is put on an alveolus, it may burst. As well as damaging the individual alveolus, this can mean that the child develops a pneumothorax, because air can be blown into the pleural space. Another problem with putting too much pressure into the alveoli is that, if they over-inflate, it can compress the tiny capillaries that run round them and allow the oxygen to be taken up and carbon dioxide to be removed. If the capillaries are squashed, then the blood cannot travel through them effectively; this means that oxygen and carbon dioxide cannot move efficiently either. Clearly, over-inflation of the alveoli is not healthy. However, as positive pressure ventilation forces air into the lungs until it achieves a set pressure, it can be hard to completely avoid this problem.

Although over-inflating the lungs is undesirable, it is important that they are inflated enough. If insufficient pressure is delivered, the alveoli do not inflate enough, and too little oxygen reaches them. It also means that the elastic recoil of the alveoli is reduced (if you stretch a piece of elastic less, it springs back less when you let go). This means that the secretions and fluid (which would usually move with the action of the elastic recoil of the alveoli) accumulate, and the risk of the child developing an infection is increased.

The pressure at the end of a breath is also important. Although the end of a breath might suggest that the alveoli are empty, as we know, this is not the case. At the end of each breath the alveoli should remain very slightly inflated, so the pressure should not go down to zero. It is usually set at about 3–5 cm H_2O. If the end pressure is set too low, the lungs empty too much, and (as well as it being harder for them to refill again) this will mean that there is less time for gas exchange to happen because the air is removed from the lungs more quickly. However, if the end pressure is set too high, this is also problematic, because the lungs do not empty well enough. This means that carbon dioxide is not removed and, because a significant amount of air remains in the lungs, new, oxygenated, air cannot replace it.

The pressures provided by ventilators therefore matter a great deal. Managing these pressures in long-term ventilation can be complicated though, because the child may already have damaged lungs. This may mean that they need more pressure than would usually be recommended both to inflate their lungs and at the end of expiration. Giving enough pressure for current need, without creating more damage or crossing the fine line between enough to be effective and too much, can be very difficult. The readings you see in most textbooks may not look like those you see on a child with long-term lung damage. If you notice this, it is advisable to find out why, in this case, things are different.

Safety issues

As well as understanding why the children you work with need a particular type of respiratory support, and the specific risks associated with different ways of providing this support, there are some practical and safety issues that you should be aware of with almost all equipment. The equipment you use will only do what it is meant to if it is working properly. If it malfunctions, it will probably not deliver the therapy it is meant to, and may harm the child.

Firstly, in order to ensure that you are alerted to any problems relating to the equipment or to the child's condition during your shift, you need to check that the alarm limits are set correctly. Machines often have default alarm limit settings; but you should check that the limits beyond which the alarms will sound are correct for the child you are caring for, and that the alarm volume is set so that you can hear it.

You also need to make sure that:

- the settings on the machine are what you expect them to be (although you should not change prescribed settings on a machine, it is important for you to check that the settings are as prescribed);
- the connections between the equipment and child are, and remain, intact (connections can become loose as well as disconnecting, and this will allow pressure and air to leak out);
- tubing is, and remains, free of any kinks or excess moisture (these would be difficult for gases to move through effectively and would alter the pressure as well as concentration of inspired gases).

It is also important to make regular observations, as described in Chapter 5, to determine whether the support the child is receiving is meeting their needs. At the start of every shift, check that you know where emergency and back-up equipment is kept, and that you can easily access this if the need arises. It is useful to have a standard 'checklist' for each child. This will ensure that you have checked everything before you begin your shift, and will make certain that every eventuality is catered for.

Equipment needs to be maintained regularly in order to remain safely functional, with a particular person having responsibility for organising the maintenance. Nevertheless, equipment may malfunction at any time, so you need to know where back-up equipment is located, as well as the processes for reporting any equipment problems, and initiating non-routine maintenance, to prevent children being left at risk from equipment which may not be working correctly. If there seems to be a problem with any of the equipment you use, it should be reported as soon as possible, and the child moved to equipment that is known to work correctly, rather than risking the wrong or sub-optimal therapy being delivered.

Although the child you work with will be stable enough to be at home, there is always the potential for their condition to change rapidly. You should therefore be aware of how to proceed if there is an unexpected, urgent, need for them to be reviewed, or if an emergency situation arises. This may include knowing how to summon emergency assistance related to equipment, medical or nursing advice or back-up.

Occasionally, adverse incidents related to equipment or care may happen, and you should be aware of how to report such events, so that there is clarity about exactly what happened, when, and what measures were put in place to maintain the child's safety. This is important so that damage or risk can be minimised, situations can be reviewed, any necessary changes to processes can be made, and lessons can be learned to prevent problems recurring.

Summary

Children may need varying degrees of assistance with their breathing for a variety of reasons, and an individual child may need different types or levels of assistance at different times. The ways in which they are assisted may include providing additional oxygen, CPAP, BiPAP, pressure support and mechanical ventilation.

Sometimes children and their families have used assisted ventilation almost since they were born, as Amelie has. However, for others it is introduced into their care at a later stage as their condition deteriorates, as has been the case for Tom, or suddenly and unexpectedly following trauma or illness, as Fateha experienced. Sometimes it is a relief for a child to have some assistance with their breathing, and to feel better. However, for a child or young person with a degenerative condition, the onset of using assisted ventilation can signal a deterioration in their condition, which represents a loss for them and their families, signals the progress of their disease, and is hard to accept. For Tom, who has Duchenne Muscular Dystrophy and whose brother has recently died from this condition, knowing that he is now at the stage of needing BiPAP is likely to create feelings of fear or sadness, as well as appreciation of any improvement in his quality of life that it brings. Individuals may therefore respond in a variety of ways to a suggestion that using assisted ventilation might be necessary or beneficial to them; and it may not always be welcome, even if its use improves their condition and quality of life.

Chapter 5

Assessing a child's respiratory status

If the child you care for has a respiratory problem, you need to assess their breathing in order to decide whether what is currently being done to assist them is effective. There are a number of machines and measurements that you can use to do this, but the most important information of all comes from assessing the child themselves.

General demeanour

One of the first and most important things to notice about a child is their general demeanour: whether they seem calm and at ease, or are a bit more irritable than usual, anxious, or cannot settle. Knowing the child and listening to what their parents tell you about them is vitally important. Often the first clues that the body is not getting quite enough oxygen, and is retaining a bit too much carbon dioxide, show as very slight signs that do not relate directly to the child's breathing, and they can be easy to miss if you do not know the child.

The parents of any child, and especially those children who have long-term health needs, often know their child better than anyone else and are experts in them, as well as their condition. They may have learned over the years that a certain sign that is ostensibly nothing to do with the child's breathing heralds a respiratory problem, and how rapidly their child can deteriorate, starting from an apparently minor change. Aisha's mother has noticed that, if Aisha starts the day with a slightly runny nose, she is likely to have become quite unwell by the evening. She has seen this on a number of occasions and, although these symptoms would, in another child, mean almost nothing, or would simply merit watching and waiting, for Aisha they herald a fairly rapid decline, and action needs to be taken. Likewise, James's mother explains that if James: '...seems a bit grumpy and on edge, probably by tomorrow he will be needing extra oxygen.'

Responsiveness

A child's level of responsiveness can be an important indicator of their respiratory status. The brain requires a significant amount of the oxygen that a child takes in, and an early sign that the brain is getting less oxygen than it needs, and has a bit too much carbon dioxide, is a child being irritable, drowsy, lacking in concentration, lethargic, or needing to sleep more but finding it hard to settle. When Tom started using BiPAP, one of the first things he noticed was that he stopped waking up feeling 'groggy' and no longer had the almost constant slight headache that he had developed.

Sometimes a child who is not getting enough oxygen is not lethargic; they are quite the opposite – very irritable, screaming, crying, refusing to lie down, because they feel as if they are struggling to breathe. Sitting quietly, playing or going to sleep are not viable options when they are very scared by this feeling. Patryc's mother recalls: 'Before he had the trache, he would get so agitated, because he was struggling to breathe. As soon as he had the trache, he was calmer, happier, easy to settle, a different baby.'

A child's level of responsiveness and behaviour can therefore be important indicators of how much oxygen they are getting and how efficiently they are getting rid of carbon dioxide. However, with some children these signs are quite hard to gauge, for example if a child has limited movement and is often unresponsive for a variety of reasons. Many children with long-term respiratory problems have plenty of reasons to feel unhappy, or be unco-operative, upset or quiet. Fateha, for example, has lost the ability to do many of the things that her peers enjoy and that she once enjoyed as well, so it is hardly surprising if from time to time she is quiet, withdrawn or angry, or feels irritable. James is quite often frustrated by wanting to do things on his own, which he needs assistance with, or when people cannot understand what he wants to say. This can mean that he gets very irritable, and has major tantrums, but they are often worse or happen more frequently and with less cause when he is slightly unwell. His mother is adept at gauging whether one of his outbursts is a regular tantrum, or something that heralds illness, but other people struggle to do this.

To put together the whole picture of what is happening with a child, you need to see what things are going on, and understand the most likely reasons for what seems to be happening. As well as looking at the way the child is responding to their environment and talking to their parents about their responses, it is important to recognise what physical signs may indicate that they are having difficulty breathing.

Respiratory rate

The child's respiratory rate is often a slightly later, but more concrete, indicator of how well they are managing to get oxygen into their body, and get rid of carbon dioxide. Counting how many times a child breathes per minute gives you an idea of whether they are trying to get more oxygen in and get rid of more carbon dioxide. If they are, they will usually, at least initially, increase their respiratory rate. To know if this is happening, you need to know what a child's normal respiratory rate should be. There are guidelines for the expected range of respiratory rates at any given age (see Table 1 below). However, these may be slightly different in a child with a long-term respiratory problem. For example, Aisha's breaths are very shallow, because her muscles do not move her ribs and diaphragm very efficiently, so she always breathes more frequently than the 'textbook rate' because her body tries to compensate for this. However, this slightly raised rate is usual for her. As well as knowing the textbook respiratory rates for children, you therefore also need to know what the expected respiratory rate is for the child you work with.

Table 1: Expected respiratory rates in children and young people

Age	Respiratory rate (breaths per minute)
Newborn	30–50
1 year	26–40
2 years	20–30
4 years	20–26
6 years	18–24
8 years	17–23
10 years	15–22
12 years	14–21
14 years	12–20
16 years	11–14

Adapted from:
J. MacGregor (2008) Introduction to the anatomy and physiology of children (2nd edition). Routledge: London and New York.

Everyone's respiratory rate falls when they go to sleep. We breathe less frequently and less deeply when we are asleep because our metabolic needs are lower and so we do not need as much oxygen. The impulses associated with 'behavioural drives', described in Chapter 3, which assist in breathing, are also much less prominent while we are asleep, so we do not breathe as frequently or as deeply (Saladin and Miller 2004). When you check a child's respiratory rate it is therefore important to note whether they are awake or asleep, as well as the number of breaths that they take.

If a child is trying to get more oxygen in, and get rid of carbon dioxide, their respiratory rate will usually increase to start with. However, as they become exhausted, their respiratory muscles tire, their body runs short of oxygen to make the respiratory muscles work, and their respiratory rate will eventually reduce because they do not have enough energy to breathe. A slowing respiratory rate in a child who has been breathing fast is not always a good sign. It may indicate that they are improving, calming down or settling, or it may signal collapse, so you need to look at more than just their respiratory rate.

A child's respiratory rate should usually be counted over a whole minute, and, as well as the number of breaths, it is useful to note whether their pattern of breathing is regular or not. The normal breathing pattern is to breathe in, have a very slight and almost unnoticeable pause, and then breathe out again, and for this pattern to continue, regularly, with about the same space between the beginning of each breath and no long gaps between breaths. Babies quite often have irregular breathing patterns, but as children get older the expectation is that they will have a fairly regular breathing pattern. If this pattern changes, it is worth noting. If a child has had an increased respiratory rate, but then develops a slow, irregular breathing pattern, with long pauses or missed breaths, they may well not be 'settling' but about to stop breathing.

Respiratory effort

As well as the rate at which a child is breathing, it is important to note how much effort they are having to make to breathe. If a child is struggling to breathe, they will often use muscles other than their intercostal and diaphragmatic muscles to try to move their ribs and diaphragm more (Sly and Collins 2006). These are often referred to as 'the accessory muscles of respiration', and they include muscles in the neck, back, shoulders and abdomen. However, babies' and small children's accessory muscles are less well developed than adults' and they cannot compensate for breathing problems in this way. Instead, when they are finding it difficult to breathe they may show nasal flaring as they attempt to reduce the resistance to airflow from their nose (Sly and Collins 2006), and develop retractions or recession.

Retractions or recession are terms used to describe the inward movement of the chest wall, which is often seen when a baby or small child tries to overcome a problem with their breathing. Because babies have very pliable chest walls, when they create a large suction pull within their chest cavity, instead of increasing their lung volume, the tissue between the ribs (intercostal), under the sternum (substernal), above the collarbone (supraclavicular) or below the trachea (suprasternal/tracheal tug) draws in as the pressure in their chest falls. You may also see 'head bobbing' as they try to breathe more deeply, and abdominal paradox (an inward movement of the child's abdominal wall as they breathe in). As children get older, their chest walls become less pliable, so these signs are not so likely to be seen. Their accessory muscles also develop, so they are better able to compensate for breathing difficulties.

All these signs may, however, be complicated in children with a long-term respiratory problem. Aisha has very poor head control, and cannot sit unaided, so it can be hard to tell if her head is 'bobbing' because of a respiratory problem, or because she has difficulty holding it in place. Tom has significant scoliosis, so although it is possible to see when he is using his accessory muscles to breathe, it is not as straightforward as it is with some other young people. When a child is in Fateha's situation, and is not able to make any respiratory effort at all, then none of these signs will be seen. This means that if Fateha's ventilator became disconnected or the settings were inadequate for her, she could not make any attempt to compensate for, or overcome this.

Another factor to consider in a child with long-term respiratory compromise is that they may have almost constant symptoms of respiratory compromise. James always has mild substernal recession and tracheal tug. It is therefore important to know if any of the signs that would usually signal compromise are the norm for a particular child, and how you would know when they had moved into a situation of danger. For example, although James has mild substernal recession and tracheal tug all the time, if this worsens, it means that fairly prompt action is required because he has very little leeway before deteriorating. This requires the staff who work with him to be very clear about the baseline from which they are working, and to know how quickly action needs to be taken if things start to change.

Chest movement

Along with noting the child's respiratory rate and effort, you also need to observe how effective their breathing is. If they are taking a large number of shallow breaths, this may mean that very little air is actually reaching the alveoli. You can assess the depth of a child's breathing by looking at their chest movement. If their chest is moving, then air is moving; if it is not moving, then air is not moving, however much effort they are making. If a child is making a great deal of effort, and is moving quite a lot in terms of accessory muscle use, recession, nasal flaring, paradoxical abdominal movements, or distress, but their chest wall and diaphragm are not moving much, then things are not going well.

Ideally, a child's chest should move equally on both sides, with the right and left side rising and falling synchronously. If it is not, it may mean that there is an obstruction somewhere. For example if Patryc's tracheostomy tube becomes slightly dislodged, the air he takes in may go preferentially to one lung; and, although both lungs may receive some air, his chest will not move evenly. If Aisha develops an infection in the lower and middle lobes of her right lung, the right side of her chest is likely to move less efficiently than the left because not as much air can get in. This might be seen as her chest wall not moving evenly on both sides. Observing this can sometimes be challenging though. Tom has quite marked scoliosis, which means that his chest wall does not move synchronously and evenly at any time. To check whether his respiratory movements are effective, it is necessary to think about the anatomy of his rib cage and diaphragm, and to look at this, rather than assessing him against generic expected chest movements. Aisha always has relatively shallow breaths, and less chest movement than another child her age would, so it is important for the staff who work with her to know the baseline that they are assessing from.

Breath sounds

If you are able to, it is useful to learn to listen for the sound of air entering and leaving the lungs using a stethoscope (auscultation). This gives you one more tool in your kit to assess a child's breathing. As well as observing whether or not the chest seems to rise and fall, you can listen to specific parts of the lung and hear whether there is good air movement there. Even if you cannot use auscultation, it is important to note the sounds a child makes when they breathe.

Snoring signals partial airway obstruction and may mean that the child has a partially occluded airway. What needs to be done about this depends on why the airway is occluded. It may simply mean that you need to reposition the child. Aisha has very poor head control, and if she is asleep in her chair and snoring it is likely to mean that she is partially obstructing her airway. As she is unlikely to be able to move her head to rectify this herself, she needs assistance. She often uses a soft neck pillow to help support her head and maintain her airway when she is dozing.

A child making a grunting sound when they breathe should alert you to the possibility that they are experiencing respiratory difficulty. Grunting is thought to be a result of a child trying to create their own version of CPAP: trying to keep their airways and alveoli open a bit longer so that more gas exchange can occur. This is likely to mean that their body knows that they need more oxygen, and is trying to get it.

Wheezing is a sound that everyone probably recognises. It is a continuous, high-pitched, whistling sound, which shows that air is trying to travel through tubes that have, for whatever reason, become narrower. When people talk about wheezing they often think of asthma, where inflammation, constriction and subsequent obstruction narrows the airways, and it's difficult for air to get through. However, wheezing can occur because of anything that causes airway obstruction. It is usually most marked when the child is breathing out (expiration), but it can also occur during inspiration, and may occur on both the inspiratory and expiratory parts of the child's breath. It is also more common in younger children, because their airways are narrower and therefore more prone to obstruction.

Stridor and wheeze can easily be confused, because stridor is also a high-pitched sound, but it is rougher than a wheeze, and sometimes described as sounding a bit like crowing. Stridor is caused by turbulent air flow in the upper airway. Like wheeze, it is commoner in younger children because they have narrower airways. It is usually more marked on inspiration, but can also occur as the child breathes out, or can be present on both inspiration and expiration. Tracheomalacia, which Patryc has, is one of the most common causes of expiratory stridor in children.

It can often be difficult to distinguish between the different sounds that may occur during breathing, especially if you are not used to listening for them. When assessing a child's breathing, it's not vital to know for certain whether they have, for example, a stridor or a wheeze. It's far more important to notice any changes from their 'normal' breathing sounds, whether they seem to occur on inspiration or expiration, and to report these changes to the appropriate person or people so that they can be further assessed and acted on.

When observing a child's breathing, you have to think about a lot more than just their respiratory rate. The respiratory rate matters, but pattern, depth, chest movement and breathing sounds are also important. In addition, there are other physiological clues that you should also consider when you are assessing how well a child is breathing.

Heart rate

If the body is low on oxygen, the heart will usually beat faster to try to get more oxygen distributed. This is a good short-term solution, but if not enough oxygen is getting in, this will soon become ineffective because, however fast the heart pumps, there is not enough oxygen available for delivery. Also, the heart itself is a muscle. As such, it needs energy to pump effectively, so it needs oxygen too. When there is not enough oxygen, there is not enough energy for the heart to do its regular job, let alone extra work. If it does not get enough oxygen, then the heart muscle can become damaged or stop working. And if the heart muscle stops working, the heart stops. So, although an increased heart rate is a useful initial response to low oxygen levels, it is not something that should be allowed to continue for long without knowing about, and acting on, the reason. The usual heart rates for children can be seen in Table 2 on page 64. However, as with a child's respiratory rate, it is important to know the usual rate for the particular child you are working with, as well as the textbook rates.

Table 2: Expected heart rates in children and young people

Age in years	Heart rate (beats per minute)
Under 1	110–160
2–5	95–140
5–12	80–120
Over 12	60–100

Adapted from:

J. MacGregor (2008) *Introduction to the anatomy and physiology of children* (2nd edition). Routledge: London and New York.

The skin

A child's skin also gives you some clues about their breathing status. The body has an order of priority in which it will let things go. The appropriately named vital organs – the heart, lungs and brain (the ones you really cannot do without) – are the most important. All things being equal, the body will preserve them at the expense of the other organs and systems. The first things that the body decides it can manage without, and also the most distant parts from the heart's pump, are the skin and the extremities (hands and feet). So, when oxygen levels begin to fall, they are the first to get a limited circulation of blood. The result of this is that the skin becomes cold, and often clammy and mottled and the child's hands and feet become cold. If a child with an otherwise normal temperature has cold hands and feet, or cold, pale and mottled skin, it can be a sign that they are not getting enough oxygen. There are of course many other reasons why a child may have cold hands and feet – for example, children who are immobile, like Fateha, often have cool feet and hands related to lack of movement – but it is something to look out for and add to the overall picture of a child's condition.

Children who are low on oxygen may also look slightly grey, especially around their lips and eyes. It is often said that a blue tinge to the skin, known as cyanosis, is a sign of low oxygen and high carbon dioxide levels. It is, but it is usually a relatively late sign in children who do not have long-term low oxygen levels. Cyanosis occurs when the blood has very high carbon dioxide levels, and for this to happen, the child's oxygen supply and removal of carbon dioxide has to be compromised for quite some time. Some children with chronic respiratory problems or heart disease are always slightly 'blue', but in a child who is otherwise well, or who is not usually cyanosed, it indicates serious compromise. Some children with long-term respiratory problems may become cyanosed more quickly than other children, because they are already running on the low end of oxygenation and the high end of carbon dioxide levels, so the step to cyanosis is not particularly great. For example, James becomes quite grey fairly quickly if he develops any respiratory problem, even a cold, and gets a blue tinge on his lips almost as soon as he gets a cough. Often, his mother will increase his oxygen as soon as he starts looking slightly grey, because she knows that he will deteriorate quite rapidly. This can be difficult for the staff who work with him, because they are not authorised to alter treatment, including oxygen delivery. That is one of the challenges of working with expert parents, and will be discussed in Chapter 7.

Feeding

The skin and extremities are the first to be deprived of oxygen, and the gut comes next. This is one of the reasons why some children with respiratory problems have difficulty absorbing their feeds, and why feed absorption can give an indication of a child's respiratory function. The gut relies on muscle movement to propel its contents. If it is deprived of oxygen, it does not have the necessary energy to move its contents along, or to absorb feeds. This means that a child who is not getting enough oxygen is unable to absorb the feeds that arrive in their stomach. At the same time, it is likely that their diaphragmatic movements and attempts to use their abdominal muscles to aid their breathing will be compressing their stomach. This creates a risk of the child vomiting and aspirating their feed into their lungs, especially if their level of consciousness is impaired.

A child has to be able to co-ordinate breathing and swallowing in order to drink and eat; and the harder it is for them to breathe, the harder it is for them to co-ordinate eating and drinking. When you look at a child who is having difficulty in breathing and watch the movement of their abdomen, it seems logical that feeding is not going to be easy for them.

Some children with long-term respiratory problems also have problems with feeding as a separate issue. One of these problems might be just manageable. But the combination of breathing problems and feeding problems creates a greater problem for the child than either would on its own. James had severe gastro-oesophageal reflux, and this in itself might have meant that he required tube feeding. However, when combined with his respiratory problems because of premature birth, the need was even greater because co-ordinating breathing and feeding was very difficult for him. Tube feeding also allowed him to be given small frequent feeds, and continuous overnight feeds, which reduced the volume of feed in his stomach at any one time, made it easier for him to absorb his feeds, and thus less likely that he would vomit and aspirate his feeds.

Kidneys

In the hierarchy of the body's organs, the kidneys go next. This can mean that a child who is low on oxygen has limited blood supply to the kidneys, and thus does not produce as much urine as usual. A falling urine output can therefore be one sign that a child is not getting enough oxygen. If they are also not feeding well, and vomiting, this will contribute to a falling urine output though, because they will not be taking in enough fluid.

The child's general demeanour, breathing, heart rate, skin, warmth of their hands and feet, ability to feed, and urine output can all be checked without any equipment at all. However, one thing that does require equipment is monitoring how well oxygen is being transported by red blood cells, using pulse oximetry.

Pulse oximetry

One very basic way of seeing how well oxygen is being transported around the body is by using pulse oximetry. This is also often referred to as oxygen saturation monitoring. Pulse oximetry gives a basic indication of how well oxygen is being delivered to tissues, but it does not tell you everything about whether the tissues are receiving enough oxygen, and does not tell you if carbon dioxide is being removed from them.

Pulse oximetry looks at how well oxygen is being transported by the red blood cells. The blood is made up of plasma, white blood cells, platelets and red blood cells. A small proportion of the oxygen that circulates around the body is carried in the plasma (and that is the oxygen level which the partial pressure of oxygen in blood gases refers to), but the majority is carried by red blood cells (haemoglobin). There are four sites within each red blood cell that are able to carry oxygen and when they are all full, that blood cell is described as being fully saturated with oxygen. The oxygen saturation percentage that you see on a pulse oximeter tells you what percentage of the body's red blood cells are saturated with oxygen. A 95% oxygen saturation reading means that the red blood cells are 95% saturated with oxygen. The usual aim is for oxygen saturation levels to be above 95% (Valdez-Lowe et al. 2009).

A pulse oximeter uses a sensor (or probe) that directs light through a pulsating capillary bed on a selected site (often the child's finger, but other sites which allow light to pass across pulsating capillary beds are equally acceptable, such as toes or ear lobes). The light uses red and infrared wavelengths and detects how much of each type of light is absorbed. Oxyhaemoglobin (haemoglobin carrying oxygen) and deoxyhaemoglobin (haemoglobin that is not carrying oxygen) absorb light differently: oxyhaemoglobin absorbs less red and more infrared light. The sensor determines the ratio of each type of light, and from this calculates the red blood cells' oxygen saturation percentage (Paragas 2008, Valdez-Lowe *et al.* 2009).

Although oxygen saturation recordings are useful, and give some indication of the child's oxygenation, they do not measure the partial pressure of gases, the haemoglobin level, or the heart's ability to pump the blood that is carrying oxygen around the body.

The oxygen saturation level and changes in this do not exactly match the partial pressure of oxygen in the plasma and changes in it. The relationship between oxygen saturation level and the partial pressure of oxygen can be represented as an s-shaped curve (called the oxyhaemoglobin dissociation curve), a diagram of which is shown in Figure 16 (below). This illustrates the relationship between the oxygen saturation level (the amount of oxygen being carried by haemoglobin) and the partial pressure of oxygen (the oxygen in the plasma portion of the blood in the arteries).

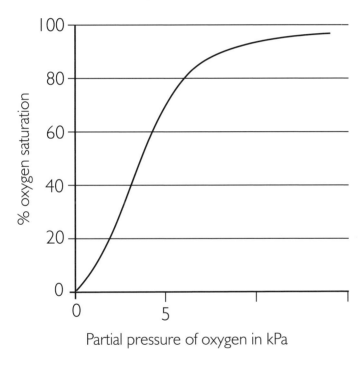

Figure 16 **The oxyhaemoglobin dissociation curve**

When the partial pressure of oxygen in arterial blood is high, the oxygen saturation reading is also high; so when one score is high, both scores are usually high. However, as the partial pressure of oxygen falls slightly, to the upper limits of normal, the oxygen saturation level hardly changes. At this point, a child's oxygen exchange in the lungs may be becoming less effective, but the oxygen saturation levels will not let you know what is happening yet. By the time a child's oxygen saturation level falls below 90%, the partial pressure of oxygen will have fallen considerably. Once the partial pressure of oxygen is below about 8 kPa, the oxygen saturation level falls suddenly, and rapidly, with even small changes in the partial pressure of oxygen (Booker 2008). This is one reason why a child may drop their oxygen saturation readings a little, appear to 'sit around' 90% for a while and then suddenly and precipitously drop their saturation readings through the 80s and 70s and lower. By the time this happens, the child has very low oxygen saturation levels, and the partial pressure of oxygen in their plasma is also very low.

Whether or not anaemia affects the accuracy of pulse oximetry readings has been debated (Valdez-Lowe *et al.* 2009). However, anaemia does affect oxygen supply to body tissue. The oxygen saturation level only shows the saturation of the red blood cells that exist. So, if a child is very anaemic then, even if all their red blood cells are fully saturated with oxygen, not enough oxygen will be delivered to the tissues because there are not enough red blood cells to carry all the oxygen the body needs. Similarly, if the heart is not pumping effectively, then not enough oxygen will be delivered to the tissues, however well saturated the individual red blood cells are with oxygen.

The oxygen saturation level therefore gives you some idea of how well oxygenated a child is, but it is not a completely accurate measurement of their oxygenation. It becomes less accurate, the lower the reading is and relatively inaccurate when the saturation level falls below 80% (Jubran 1999, Booker 2008). However, it is a useful rough guide.

For oxygen saturation monitoring equipment to work well, the probe site must be clean and dry so that the light sources can work effectively. If the probe is not well positioned, is not well secured, or if the child is moving, the measurements made by oxygen saturation monitors may be inaccurate because these things make it more difficult for the probe to detect the different absorptions of light (Paragas 2008, Valdez-Lowe *et al.* 2009). If the blood supply to the area where the probe is positioned is poor, then the reading will probably be inaccurate because the probe is designed to measure pulsing capillary blood (Paragas 2008, Valdez-Lowe *et al.* 2009). For example, if a child has an oxygen saturation probe on their foot, and their foot is cold, and has reduced blood supply, the reading may well be difficult to obtain or be inaccurate. In addition, for the monitor to alert you appropriately to any problems, the alarms have to work and be set to the correct limits.

When children have long-term respiratory problems, the same basic principles of oxygen saturation monitoring apply as they do to all children. However, their baseline oxygen saturation level may not be as high as one would expect. For example, James rarely has an oxygen saturation level above 92%. Some children with long-term respiratory problems or cardiac problems have, as their normal oxygen saturation reading, a level that would usually mean that their partial pressure of oxygen was very low and their oxygen saturation readings were about to go into a sharp decline. However, because this is the usual level for them, the expected rapid deterioration does not occur. It may, nonetheless, mean that if their oxygen saturation level does start to fall it will fall very rapidly, without giving you the thinking time that you might have when another child's oxygen saturation readings began to drop.

Summary

When you are assessing a child's respiratory status, the first and most important thing to do is to look at the child, and see how they are – their general demeanour and position. You should also check their respiratory rate, pattern and depth, listen for any unusual respiratory sounds, check their heart rate, skin colour and temperature, and look at their feeding and urine output. It is also often useful to be able to check their oxygen saturation level. Remember that the information gained from a monitoring device will only be as good as the person using the device and their knowledge and interpretation of the information presented. Monitoring devices do not replace expert observation, but they can be very useful in terms of providing additional information and measurable data.

Once you have all this information, you need to put it all together, and combine it with your knowledge of the child themselves, and the information their parents give you, to make a decision about what should happen next.

Chapter 6
Discharge planning

When it becomes clear that a child who is in hospital will need long-term respiratory support, a great deal of planning is often required to enable them to go home (Department of Health 2004b). Understanding the complexity of what has to be arranged can help you to contribute effectively to this process if you are involved in it. Even if you are not involved in the discharge process, it may still be useful for you to understand what has happened prior to children being able to come home, and the sometimes difficult decisions that families and service providers have had to make to achieve this. Fateha's mother comments:

> 'When we were planning how we could bring Fateha home, there were so many things I had to think about, and it was sometimes hard to decide what was best, for everyone. Sometimes people say to me: "Why didn't you do this?" or "Did you not think of doing that?" Although they are trying to be helpful, these are often decisions I can't change now, and it's easy to be wise with hindsight. I did what seemed best at the time, most of my decisions were made after a lot of hard soul-searching, and it can be hurtful to have them criticised by people who weren't there at the time and don't know everything I was trying to balance.'

Arranging a child's discharge from hospital can be a protracted process, and delays should be kept to the minimum. It is, nonetheless, also important that enough time is taken to ensure that the right arrangements are in place, and that, as far as possible, every eventuality planned for. If a child goes home before everything is really ready, it is often problematic in the long term for them, their families, and those who support them. Amelie's mother recalls:

> 'When we were organising getting her home from hospital, we were so desperate to get out of hospital, and be a family again, that it was tempting to go before everything was really finalised, and just muddle through, for the sake of being home, until things got up and running. I was given a really good piece of advice though, and I'm glad I followed it.

Another mum said to me: "If it's not set up before you go, the chances of it happening once you're home are much slimmer, and it will take even longer to get everything you need organised once you're out of hospital." So we held out, and I'm glad we did. It meant waiting a few extra weeks, which at the time seemed like forever, but it meant that everything really was ready when we got home.'

In order to make effective plans for a child's discharge from hospital, a comprehensive assessment needs to be made of what their needs will be once they are at home, and what support they and their family will require. If their needs are not fully and accurately assessed, the support they are provided with will probably not be ideal. The assessment should include: what the child's physical needs are; what medical supplies and equipment they will need at home; what their social, emotional and educational needs are, and how these can be met; and the needs of other members of the family.

Equipment and supplies

An essential part of planning a child's discharge from hospital is determining what medication and other prescribed items (such as feeds) they will require; what supplies they will need (for example, suction catheters, ventilator circuits, feeding equipment); how and when supplies and prescription items will be ordered and delivered (for example, it may be important to check that the family will not be expected to wait in every day in order to take deliveries of different items). The supplies that children need may be bulky, and consideration will have to be given to the space that families have to accommodate them. It is also useful to establish at the outset what back-up plans exist in case supplies unexpectedly run low, or there is additional demand – for example, for holidays. Having these arrangements agreed on before they are required may make it less problematic to put them in place quickly if they are needed.

Firstly, the equipment a child will require to meet their respiratory needs, and any other equipment (for instance, mobility aids, hoists, etc.) needs to be established. This includes determining not just what they will need, but whether the proposed equipment will be functional and will assist them in their home environment, rather than creating further challenges for the family.

It is also important that the child has access to equipment that will enable them to leave the house for social activities, and to attend school, with the minimum difficulty. It is useful to explore whether equipment, particularly equipment that is bulky or difficult to transport, can be duplicated in more than one location. For example, it may be possible to make standing frames, feed pumps and oxygen concentrators available both at home and at the child's school, as they will be difficult for parents to bring in every day. James's mother explains:

> 'I am already planning for when James goes to school, and one thing I am aiming for is to get them to agree to have a frame, seating system and oxygen concentrator that we can leave at the school. I know I may be pushing my luck, but if I have to carry all that in every day, plus everything else he needs, and push his chair, and get Alice into her class, I just can't see how I will do it.'

Accommodation

When a child requires long-term respiratory support, their family home may no longer meet their needs. In some cases, houses require adaptations to be made, or families may have to relocate to accommodate the child's needs (Margolan *et al.* 2004). In this situation, they may not only need assistance to plan their accommodation so as to best meet the child's needs and the needs of other family members, but also to plan for the long term as well as the short term, especially if their child's needs are likely to increase as they get older. This can be difficult for families to consider, especially when they are still getting used to the idea of their child having long-term health needs. However, it is often beneficial in the long term, to avoid the need to undertake repeated housing adaptations or relocations (Hewitt-Taylor 2007).

Guiding families about what other families have found helpful, and putting them in touch with families who are in similar situations, may be useful, to help them to think about every eventuality, and make decisions that best meet their needs in both the short and long term. Some resources of this type are suggested in Box 3 (page 74. James's mother describes how:

> 'The other day I was talking online to a mum whose baby is waiting to come home from the neonatal unit. She needs oxygen, like James, and it sounds as if she is going to have long-term mobility problems. The woman I was chatting to was saying that she was desperate to get home but she needs to move, because they are in a one-bedroom flat. She said she had found this two-bedroom flat that would probably be OK, and I said to her: "Don't just think of now, when all you'll have to do is lug the oxygen and a baby in a buggy. If you're moving, think of later on, when you may still need oxygen, but you may also have a wheelchair, and everything, including your daughter, will be heavier and harder to move. Think of small things, like: are there any little steps here and there, which will become difficult to manage as she gets older? Otherwise, you could end up moving again or getting ramps put in, in a couple of years' time."'

Box 3: Peer support groups for parents

Our-Kids: a group of parents, caregivers and others who work with children with disabilities and developmental delays

http://www.our-kids.org/

Parents of disabled children

http://www.parentsofdisabledchildren.co.uk

Special Kids in the UK: a charity that offers advice, information and support for the families of children with special needs

http://www.specialkidsintheuk.org/

Staffing

Assessing the child's needs includes: considering what their physical care requirements will be; how much assistance their parents need and would like to have with this; and how this will best be organised around the family's lifestyle and priorities. Finding the right level of input, which will be beneficial for the child and family, should be the goal – neither too little, nor too much. Having a child who requires long-term respiratory support creates a significant workload for their parents. But effective support usually involves finding a balance between families having adequate assistance and also enough privacy and time alone with their child. In addition, because budgets are finite and demand almost infinite, it may be necessary to prioritise what families most want, as well as what they would ideally like if resources were unlimited. Again, it is sometimes useful for them to talk to other families in similar situations about their experiences, to enable them to gain as much perspective as they can on what arrangements are likely to be helpful, workable and realistic.

Recruiting staff to provide for a child's day-to-day care needs is often an essential part of the discharge process, and may not be easy to achieve. Although there are an increasing number of children who require long-term respiratory support, the number of staff available in each local area remains relatively small. This means that in some cases there may not be a bank of staff who are readily available and trained to undertake this type of work. Staff therefore often need to be appointed and trained for each individual child, and this can take time and significantly delay a child's discharge home (Margolan *et al.* 2004). Amelie's mother recalls:

'I was amazed at how long it took to get staff. You have this delusion, because until you have to you never think about it, that there are staff out there, ready to work with you, but there aren't. We had to wait about five extra weeks because one girl who they had appointed changed her mind. They had to find someone else, and train her up, before we could go home. Luckily they found someone fairly quickly, who didn't have to give notice in the job they were in, or else it would have taken even longer.'

Short break services

It is important to give parents opportunities to have some time off from their role as carers (Department of Health 2004b, MacDonald and Callery 2004, Heaton *et al.* 2005, Yantzi *et al.* 2006). Other parents can often get breaks from childcare by using grandparents or friends, but this is less likely to be an option for parents whose children require long-term respiratory support (Yantzi *et al.* 2006). Whether short break services will be helpful and available should therefore be considered in discharge planning.

The reality is often that short break care is not easily available (Margolan *et al.* 2004), and although families may, at the point of discharge, not feel that this is something they need, they may be well advised to consider it as a useful long-term option. James's mother comments:

'I would advise anyone going home to ask for short break care. I don't remember being asked, and when you're in hospital, you probably feel as if you don't need it, or want it, because you just want to get home. But as time goes on, you don't get a break, to just be on your own, or with your other child. When your child is on oxygen you can't say to your mum: "Can he come to you overnight?" Once you're home, and coping, it is harder to get it agreed, and short break services are like hen's teeth round here. So I would say, ask for it, and ask early, because when the time comes, you will appreciate it.'

Specialist input

As well as the staff who provide their day-to-day healthcare, children who need long-term respiratory support will usually also have input from a number of members of the multidisciplinary team. For their support to work effectively, everyone involved in their care needs to be aware of the input of other individuals and organisations, so that there are no gaps and no unnecessary duplication in provision. Because of the range of professionals involved in a child's care, it is often useful for the family to have a named Key Worker who acts as a central point of contact, and as a co-ordinator for all the parties involved (Department of Health 2004b, Boddy *et al.* 2006, Greco *et al.* 2006).

Some of the staff who are likely to be involved in supporting children and their families are listed below.

Specialist nurses

These are registered nurses who have experience and additional training in a specific area – for example, a respiratory nurse specialist or a tracheostomy nurse specialist. Their role is to provide specific and specialist input and advice for the child, family and others involved in providing their day-to-day care.

Community children's nurses

These are registered children's nurses with a community nursing qualification, who have direct involvement with children's care. Depending on how the individual child's care is organised, community children's nurses may therefore: provide for and co-ordinate their day-to-day care needs; act as their Key Worker; provide specific input, or oversee the support that another agency is primarily providing (for example, if a private healthcare organisation is commissioned to provide the child's day-to-day care, under the direction of the Primary Care Trust's children's services).

Medical staff

The medical staff involved in the child's care are likely to include their general practitioner, a range of hospital-based specialists and a community paediatrician. When a child is being discharged from hospital, there should be a clear plan as to how the input from hospital-based specialists will continue, and how their input will be co-ordinated with medical staff, nursing staff and allied health professionals in the community. Families should also be clear about which medical staff they should contact in different situations, and who is their first port of call in an emergency.

Physiotherapists

A physiotherapist's main role is to identify and maximise movement potential, including chest movement, and thus they are likely to have some involvement with most children who require long-term respiratory support. The child may see physiotherapists who are both hospital- and community-based.

Occupational therapists

Occupational therapists focus on using specific, purposeful activities to prevent disability and promote independent function in all aspects of daily living. Children with long-term respiratory problems are likely to have input from occupational therapists to assist them and their families in designing activities, and selecting assistive devices and adaptations that will assist them at home, in school, and any other location. It is likely that children will have input from hospital-based and community-based occupational therapists, and may have school-based occupational therapy.

Dieticians

Children who have additional nutritional needs, such as difficulty in feeding or assisted feeding, are likely to have input from a dietician.

Speech and language therapists

Children who have additional communication needs, and those who have difficulty swallowing, will often have input from a speech and language therapist.

Ambulance services and paramedics

Children who require long-term respiratory support may not require input from ambulance services or paramedics. However, it is useful for these services to be aware of them and their needs, so that if they become acutely unwell, or require ambulance input, the staff who visit them are aware of their baseline needs, and familiar with any specific requirements they have. Patryc's mother explains:

> 'We have never needed to call an ambulance, but I was advised to make sure the hospital had contacted the ambulance service so that if we did ever need to call one they knew that Patryc had a trache, and were happy to deal with it. We had two paramedics come and see us in hospital, so they knew what to do, just in case, and knew that if they got a call to our address, there was a child with a trache.'

Social workers

Children who require long-term respiratory support are likely to have, or have access to, a social worker. The social worker's role includes assessing the child's and family's needs and determining what services and support they need from a social perspective. This may include: advocacy, liaison with other agencies, financial and benefits advice, housing advice, referral to local authorities for aids and adaptations, referral to relevant charities, short break care, and assistance with home care.

Education services

A child's discharge plan should encompass how their education needs, including pre-school and school provision, will be met. This may include which placement they intend to access, what support they will need, and by which agency this will be provided. Some of their assistance may be provided by healthcare or social care services, but some may be the responsibility of the education service. Regardless of who is responsible for providing specific aspects of the child's support, their classroom teacher, classroom assistants, and the school Special Educational Needs Co-ordinator (SENCO) and, where relevant, the appropriate pre-school placement staff will all need to be considered in their discharge planning. The Local Authority is responsible for ensuring that children's educational needs, including pre-school education, are identified promptly, assessed accurately and matched with appropriate provision. This includes assessing children using statutory assessments and reviews such as Statements of Special Educational Need.

Funding

Reaching agreement on how and by whom a child's needs will be funded is an important part of planning their discharge. Whilst it is important to see the child and family holistically, funding is often provided via different sources – for example, from social care, healthcare and education budgets. Unless these sources work together, gaps can be left in provision, or there may be delays whilst agreement is reached on who will fund what.

The services that children who require long-term respiratory support need are often provided by the organisations who fund them – for example, nursing care by the Primary Care Trust, social care by Social Services, and so on. This type of provision is organised in various ways – for instance, by a Children's Community Nursing team providing the child's day-to-day care, by a specialist part of this team providing it, or by the service being contracted to another provider such as a private company.

Whilst services are often arranged in this way, it is now possible for families to exercise more choice and control than was traditionally possible over how their day-to-day support is provided, by using Direct Payments, Individual Budgets or Personal Health Budgets (DoH 2003, DoH 2009, DoH 2011). This approach to providing services has a longer history in social care than in healthcare. Direct Payments were introduced into social care through the Community Care Act (Direct Payments) (HMSO 1996). These are monetary payments made by local councils to individuals who have been assessed as needing certain services, and they are intended to give individuals choice and control over whom they employ to assist them, and when the assistance is provided (DoH 2003).

Individual Budgets were piloted in social care between 2006 and 2007 (DoH 2009). They provide individuals with information on what support they have been assessed as needing and the budget that has been set for this, to enable them to make choices about how it is provided. Individual Budgets further develop the ideal created by Direct Payments, by enabling individuals to make decisions about the exact nature and design of the support they have been assessed as needing across a range of areas. For example, Individual Budgets give people greater choice about the equipment they purchase, rather than focusing on how and by whom personal care is provided, as was often the case with Direct Payments. Using an Individual Budget, the person concerned may: manage the funds allocated to them themselves (or by a parent on their child's behalf); have them managed on their behalf by a voluntary organisation or Independent Living Trust; or leave their day-to-day management in the hands of Social Services, but use their knowledge of the 'notional sum' within which they can make choices to request the provision that best suits their needs.

Direct Payments or Individual Budgets were not traditionally available in healthcare because it was not clear whether it was legally permissible to devolve monies directly to individuals. There was also an argument that such arrangements ran counter to the principle of care provided by the National Health Service being free at the point of delivery. However, with the increasing use of such approaches in social care, a pilot of Personal Health Budgets involving Primary Care Trusts in England is now underway, and will run until 2012 (DoH 2011). Personal Health Budgets work on the same principle as Individual Budgets, but address the amount of money that is spent on meeting the health needs of a person with a long-term illness or disability. Like Individual Budgets, they may involve: a notional budget, where the NHS continues to hold the funds allocated for service provision and buys or provides the goods and services the individual has chosen; a situation where a third-party organisation that is legally independent of both the individual and the NHS (for example, an Independent User Trust or a voluntary organisation) holds the money on the person's behalf, and buys or provides the goods and services they have chosen; or a situation in which the money is transferred to the individual concerned, who buys the goods and services that they have been assessed as needing.

Whilst many families appreciate the opportunity to exercise more choice about the support they receive, using these types of approaches also creates some additional work and responsibility (Scourfield 2005). Parents who are involved in managing their child's budget may be responsible for: employing staff; making sure that they have adequate staffing cover for every shift; ensuring employment regulations are adhered to; providing annual leave, sick leave and maternity leave for their employees; purchasing equipment and ensuring that it is maintained; and organising staff training. As well as deciding whether they wish to manage their budget themselves, or have a third party such as an Independent Living Trust manage it for them, recipients of this type of funding can get assistance in managing their own budgets. This may include assistance with the practicalities of employment and information on legal aspects of employment, advocacy and advice services (DoH 2003, Glendinning *et al.* 2008). When families have opted for, or are exploring the option of, Individual Budgets or Personal Health Budgets, discharge planning may involve working with them on ensuring that they have adequate support for the day-to-day administration and management of their budget.

Fateha's mother has considered having both an Individual Budget and a Personal Health Budget for her daughter. She summarises the arguments as follows:

'I have looked into the possibility of using Individual and Personal Health Budgets for Fateha because then I could choose what we need, and when, and could hire the staff I want, and decide what I can save on so we can do something special sometimes, or get a particular piece of equipment and go without something else. The thing that puts me off is the administration and the responsibility. Now, if someone goes off sick, the PCT have to find me another person. Even if they use an agency and it's someone I am not too keen on, it's their job to do the chasing and find someone. I'm not sure I want that responsibility, and the extra work and worry of what will happen if I can't cover it. I think maybe because I have 24-hour care, I know I am covered all day every day, so I'm not so fussed about timings and things, but for people who have gaps in care provision, it would probably be good to be able to choose exactly when you have cover, so you can fit it in with the rest of your family as well.'

James's mother explains her point of view:

'I am looking very carefully at what happens with the Personal Health Budgets, because I would be really interested in that. At the moment I get night care, and I get the hours that the Home Care Team work. That means they start at eight and they leave at eight. I get the number of nights agreed, at those times. Sometimes it would be nice to be a bit more flexible, maybe to say: "Actually I don't need anyone till half past nine, and they can finish at seven." Then, with the extra two and a half hours a day I saved, I could have an extra night of cover every week. I would really like more flexibility to look at what would suit us better, within the same hours, but tailored to my family. So if Personal Health Budgets are here to stay, I will definitely be looking into that.'

Preparing parents for discharge

Although discharge plans often focus on the equipment, supplies and services that families need, and the training that staff require, parents also have to learn the skills required to manage their child's care at home. Even when they have been in hospital for some time, and have become familiar with the care their child needs, it can be very different and daunting for them to carry this out at home, where trained staff and support services are not immediately available if they experience problems. A part of the discharge process is making sure that parents are as confident as possible in managing their child's needs, in the context of their home environment, and know who to contact in case of difficulties, emergencies or changes in the child's condition.

James's mother recalls:

'When I got home, where I had been desperate to be, it was suddenly like: "Oh ... I'm on my own now. What if something happens?" Doing his feeds, I was much more nervous than I had been in hospital. I'd been doing his feeds in hospital for months, but suddenly I was aware that if he choked, or had a major seizure or something, I had no one to shout for. So it was quite scary, even though I had been doing all his care for months.'

It is useful for parents to go out with their child, to their home or in the community, before being finally discharged. This not only helps them gain confidence in the physical aspects of their child's care outside the hospital environment, but also helps them to be aware of possible challenges, pitfalls or unexpected considerations, which would be difficult to plan for. Fateha's mother recalls:

'The first time I went on a trip out from the hospital with Fateha, I was stunned by the way people looked at me, and her – the pity, the avoiding us, the stares. It was just a shock, because I had been with her in the protected hospital environment. It was useful to go on trips out to get used to doing all her care away from hospital, but also to steel myself for the way people behave, and to be able to go back to where we felt safe, even though I was desperate to get out of there, to recover from the way that made me feel. By the time we went home, I was used to it, as far as you ever are. But realising what it would be like before we were out there on our own helped me.'

Summary

Planning for the discharge home of a child who requires long-term respiratory support involves considering a wide range of services and arrangements. These include: the supplies and equipment the child will need, their accommodation, the care and support they will require, short break care options, their education and social options, their care at home, and how the range of staff who assist in meeting their needs can be sure that they communicate effectively so that service provision is not fragmented. Governance frameworks and processes will also need to be in place and agreements will have to be reached about which services will provide funding for each aspect of support, and how this will be organised. This can all take a considerable length of time, and can be frustrating for both families and staff (Margolan et al. 2004). However, when planning discharge, it is vital to encourage parents not to allow their understandable desire to be at home prevent them from gaining as full as possible an appreciation of, and preparation for, the years ahead.

As well as developing practical skills and knowledge, parents need to be given the chance to consider, and be supported in, accommodating the emotional workload of caring for their child at home. In addition, although the child's needs are those that are primarily being planned for, good discharge planning, like all types of care, should place their needs within the context of their family. It should consider how their needs impact on others, especially their siblings, and support should be organised so as to maintain a good quality of life for the other children, as well as for the child in question.

These considerations are important at the time when a child's package of support is first designed. But they are equally important throughout these children's lives, as their needs and support mechanisms change and are reviewed, and provision is developed and redesigned.

Chapter 7

Principles of working in the home setting

When children have long-term respiratory problems that require day-to-day intervention, they may not be able to live at home unless their families receive some assistance from health and social care professionals. The amount, duration and type of support required will vary, but it will always mean that families have a visitor, or visitors, in their home on a regular basis. Whilst this is necessary, it often creates challenges for all concerned. Whilst families need assistance in the home, they would probably prefer to be able to manage alone. This can mean that, whilst the help you provide is welcome, the need for this assistance (and by association, your presence) can cause difficulties for the family, or even be resented. Sometimes the most difficult part of working with children and their families is trying to provide the care and support they need, whilst minimising your intrusion into their lives.

Keeping intrusion to the minimum

Often you will meet the family you are going to work with before their child leaves hospital, when their care package is being planned. However, this is not always the case, and if you are joining an established care package, or if a child's needs have changed so that they need more care, your first meeting with the family may be in their home. Some families employ their staff directly (for example, through Personal Budgets) but staff are often appointed to work with families by service providers, without the family being directly involved. It is easy to imagine that having someone whom they have never met, or have only met briefly, allocated as a regular visitor to their home can be daunting, and anxiety provoking, for families.

On a practical level, families may feel the need to maintain a higher than usual level of tidiness and cleanliness in their homes because of staff being there, not because this creates an environment that they enjoy living in (Hewitt-Taylor 2007). Aisha's mother feels that time that she would really like to spend with her children is taken up in preparing for the carers to arrive, and making sure that the house, and in particular Aisha's room, is clean and tidy every evening.

Another practical issue for families who have support at home is that many houses are not large enough to easily accommodate the child's needs, equipment and additional adults. Amelie's parents had expected their daughters to share a room, but this was not possible because Amelie requires assisted ventilation and carers at night. Initially her parents converted their own room into Amelie's room, and slept downstairs, but this was not sustainable, so they moved house. When they moved, they gave a lot of consideration to how they could accommodate Amelie's carers so that their intrusion on the family would be reduced to a minimum. Amelie's mother explains:

> 'We got a place with an extra loo, just next to Amelie's room, because if we are all getting up and ready for school and work in the morning it means that we can use the main bathroom and the carers can use the other bathroom. We all need to get up and showered and ready, and it is nice to know that you can just fall out of the bedroom and into the bathroom without wondering if someone you have only met a few times is in the corridor waiting. Amelie's room is just slightly away from the other rooms, at the end of the corridor, and the staff have what was a small box room just next to Amelie's room, with a kettle, tea and coffee and microwave and a small fridge, so they can sit and have a drink and write their reports in peace once Amelie is awake, and I can go to the kitchen and grab a coffee without having to stop and chat or get dressed first. Juliette can go and get her breakfast without having to feel she needs to be presentable, and if she has a friend over to stay, they can slob around. It makes life much more bearable for us all. They have some privacy and so do we. We were lucky though because our parents both helped us financially so we could afford it. A lot of people couldn't.'

Having carers in the home can impact on family relationships. Arguing, expressing affection, or simply chatting with one's partner or children is likely to be overheard, which can make it almost impossible for families to have relaxed relationships and intimacy. Even telephone conversations can very rarely be guaranteed to be completely private (Hewitt-Taylor 2007). All a family's personal and business transactions may therefore be perceived as being open to scrutiny, notice or judgment. James has a carer with him five nights a week, because of his oxygen needs. This means that on those nights his mother can sleep, knowing that someone will hear and respond if his oxygen levels fall or if his nasal prongs become dislodged. However, it took her a while to get used to the carer being there. She often gets telephone calls from family or friends after

James is in bed, and on the nights she has a carer she feels she has to be more circumspect in what she says, because she can be overheard. Fateha's mother recalls that when she was arranging her finances, following her husband's death, she often discussed her situation on the telephone, and was aware that the staff who were caring for Fateha could probably overhear these conversations.

If a child needs a carer with them at night, their parents may feel a lack of privacy when they sleep, and in their bedrooms, particularly if staff sometimes have to seek advice from them during the night. Some parents describe installing call bells or intercoms so that staff do not need to visit their rooms (Hewitt-Taylor 2007). Even so, depending upon the design of the house, and how well individuals sleep, some people find that the slightest action by staff at night, and even the awareness that someone else is awake in their house, disrupts their sleep (Hewitt-Taylor 2007).

Families may also feel that they have nowhere completely private to explore or give vent to their emotions (Brett 2004). Whilst staff may be a source of emotional support, some individuals prefer to work through their feelings alone. And in such cases, having someone constantly in their home may be problematic. Tom's parents have found his deteriorating condition very difficult to deal with, especially following as it does on the death of their older son. His mother has commented that, whilst she appreciates that staff want to support them, she is a very private person and does not want to discuss how she feels, especially as few of the staff who work with Tom knew her other son. It can be difficult to know when to offer support, and when to leave people to manage alone. One of the most vital skills, when working with children who have long-term respiratory problems, is the ability to note cues from parents and children which indicate that they want to talk, be listened to, talk about something mundane instead of something emotive, or have complete privacy.

Staff visiting a house on a regular basis can mean that visitors or neighbours become aware that someone in the family has a health problem (Hewitt-Taylor 2007). Whilst this is inevitable, it means that the family's life and business is not as private as it might otherwise be. Amelie's parents have commented that the people who recently moved in next door to them seem 'desperate' to know why they have someone calling round every night. Because Amelie does not need any intervention during the day, the presence of carers at night, and occasional supplies arriving, is what suggests to the outside world that there is something different about the family.

Some families may feel that every aspect of their home and life is under scrutiny, and that observations, comments or questions about their home or lifestyle are intrusive, even if made as a part of casual conversation. For other families, such comments and questions convey an interest that they appreciate. Families' preferences about their relationship with staff, and the way in which they want them to be involved in their home and life, will be very individual and it can be difficult to note cues about this, and strike the right balance for each family (Hewitt-Taylor 2007).

Negotiation

Making sure that things run as smoothly as possible, minimising your intrusion on the family, and developing good working relationships with them all require a great deal of negotiation. There are likely to be both formal negotiations between families and service providers, and ongoing and informal day-to-day negotiations between you and the family you work with about almost every aspect of your work. The formal negotiations, which are a part of setting up the care package, may include: which aspects of the child's care and support the staff will take on, the hours that staff will work, the expectations each party may have of the work environment, and safety. However, although these aspects may appear to cover most aspects of your work, the specifics of each day's events often still have to be negotiated, such as the role you play in the family's life, and what will constitute the day-to-day 'house rules'. Aisha's parents have signed an agreement that the carer's role is purely care, not any housework or cleaning. Although this is quite clear, one of her carers comments:

'It seems very straightforward, but there are small things you have to watch out for: stacking the dishwasher, we put our stuff in and sometimes while you're waiting for the kettle to boil, you just think: "Oh, I'll stack the dishwasher for everyone", because you would just automatically do that, without it being your job, but then you think: "But if I do it once, will it become my job?" In one care package I worked in, it was those little things that in the end caused so much friction, so I am really tuned in to thinking about, and being clear about, all that stuff.'

It is often necessary to renegotiate the roles taken on by, and relationships between, staff and families – for instance, as the child's condition and age change; or as their parents become more confident in their care, as they become more exhausted by their workload, or need to have more time with their other children. The division of roles and responsibilities between staff and families may also change as families become more accustomed to their situation, and to working with staff. This can mean that the process of working together requires ongoing, sometimes almost daily negotiation, often at a very informal level. One of Fateha's carers comments:

'At first her mum was quite unsure, you know, not that she didn't trust us, but she didn't seem to think she should leave us, like it was her duty to be there, but then she gradually started saying "OK if I just pop out?" and now it's "I'm going out with Farid now, you've got my number…", which is good, because he needs his mum to himself sometimes.'

Although negotiation is often a daily part of your work, it is rare for you to be negotiating with families on a completely equal footing. Families are not usually negotiating from a position of complete choice, because their choice would generally be not to need care staff at all (Ronayne 2001, Hewitt-Taylor 2007). This may mean that they feel beholden to you or the organisation you work for, and this can make it difficult for them to state their needs. Conversely, they may feel that they have to justify what they need, which can sometimes make them appear demanding. James's mother recalls that initially she was told that she would not be entitled to support at home because James 'only needed oxygen'. She had to explain that this meant that she could not sleep at night because she was constantly woken by his oxygen saturation monitor, or feed pump. She says:

> 'I had to really be quite demanding, saying: "I need to sleep at night so I can look after him and his sister in the daytime." I'm sure they thought I was rude and demanding, but I had to be, to get what I needed, for James and his sister's sake as well as my own. Sometimes now I can feel myself bristling if I think anyone is suggesting I don't need the staff at night.'

In some instances, families may feel unable to assert their preferences and negotiate with staff, of whatever grade, for fear that they may lose the help they have, however flawed it may be. James's mother describes how:

> 'You feel that because it took so long to get staff, and because they seemed to be quite grudgingly given, if you say that one isn't doing their job, you'll just go without. Or if you upset them, they'll leave and you'll have no one. I had one who always left a mess. Not just in his room, she never washed her things up, not just cups, she'd have her cereal and toast, and leave the plates in the sink, and she'd sometimes have a meal at night and leave the plate from that too. One morning I got up and found not just her plates, but half of her meal, which she had not even left on the sink but under James's bed. It wasn't as if he had been ill that night and she hadn't had time to tidy up. But you feel that's petty, and at least you got some sleep, so leave it. But it is annoying, when someone doesn't even respect your house.'

Equally though, it can be intimidating for you to have to negotiate with confident or apparently demanding parents, because you have to work in the family's home and are probably reluctant to create tension in your workplace. On other occasions it may be difficult for you to clarify your role because you do not want to upset the family. One of Aisha's carers explains:

> 'We work until eight. I know her mum has the other two to get ready for school in the morning, and has to take Aisha on the school run with her, and it must be hard, but she is almost never ready to take over from us. We always have to emphasise that we are

going, and I am usually five or ten minutes late getting away. I do sympathise with her, and you don't want to seem petty, and create bad feeling, but I get away late almost every day because she's not quite ready.'

One part of addressing these difficult issues can be to have clear and established boundaries, for both parties to be clear about what is expected, and what is not, and to adhere to this from the outset. It is quite easy to gradually let things slip, and then have difficulty getting back to what was agreed. James's mother recalls:

'With the one who left things lying around, I had a new girl start and I heard this one saying: "Oh, she is really easy-going, you know, just make yourself at home," and I thought "Oh. Now it's going to be hard to start this one off on the right footing."'

Respect

Respect between yourself and the people whose home you work in is essential in order for you to provide them with effective support, and to have a good work environment yourself. When you work in someone's home, you need to not only respect them, but also their surroundings, personal belongings and others around them. Respecting a child and family also means being non-judgmental about their values and beliefs, and developing, finding, or agreeing on, a common value system within which everyone can work.

Being non-judgmental means that individuals and families should not be judged according to your personal standards or opinions; you do not need to pretend to be unaware of, or deny, the differences between yourself and the families you work with. That would be unrealistic, because we all have slightly different values and opinions. Being non-judgmental means being aware of your own opinions, values and beliefs, how these differ from those of others, and the effect that this could have on your work, so as to avoid these differences having a negative impact on the support you provide (Koh 1999).

This can be difficult when you work closely with families and regularly provide a great deal of direct care for their child, especially when you have different views relating to childcare practices. Being cared for by people with vastly differing values can be problematic for the child as well, in terms of consistency of expectations, rules, norms and practices. Whilst it is unlikely that many individuals will be in complete accord on all aspects of childcare, it is important to find a value system and a set of childcare practices that everyone agrees to abide by. As parents have responsibility for their child 24 hours a day, the parents' values should take priority (unless, for some reason, these are not in the child's best interests). Your task is to support families in caring for their child, not to impose your value systems on them. James's mother states:

'I have two children, and as far as possible I treat them the same, in terms of how they are allowed to behave and so on. So it is important that the carers respect my rules, because James can't be following a different set of rules from Alice, because that wouldn't be fair.'

Although your remit is to provide support for families in caring for their child, in most cases you are not employed to provide unsolicited advice on general childcare issues. This can be a very sensitive area, and you should be aware that parents' childcare practices may be subject to comments and advice that are unrelated to their child's medical or technical needs, and which would not be made if they did not require assistance with their child's health needs. Unless this is within your specific remit, or parents specifically ask your advice, giving unsolicited advice or opinions on their childcare practices may be seen as intrusive and insulting. All parents have slightly different approaches to childcare, and, unless these are harmful to the child, it is not your place to try to impose your views on them (Farasat and Hewitt-Taylor 2007). Nevertheless, whilst those who have parental responsibility for a child have the right to bring them up according to their values, priorities, beliefs and culture, there may be situations where this is harmful to the child, and you have a duty of care to every child with whom you work. The child's safety and best interests override all other considerations, and the assertion that parents' rights should be respected does not mean that you can neglect protecting children. There should be very clear mechanisms through which you can seek support and discuss any childcare practices that cause you concern.

There may also be situations where you accept a family's rules and norms but feel unable to be involved in them yourself. You should not be judgmental of families, but neither are you obliged to be in situations in which your values are not respected. For instance, there may be times when it is necessary to have a discussion involving your manager or another independent individual to enable you to work together with the child and family, and agree on a way in which you can support them without compromising your own values. One of Tom's carers comments:

'His sister really doesn't like us being there. I can understand she is grieving for her brother, and Tom is getting worse, and her parents are tied up in that, and we are in her space, but I will not be spoken to rudely. Regardless of how she is allowed to behave by her family, if she swears at me, I tell her off. One time her dad heard her swear at me, and he said nothing, so I told her that I don't mind what she thinks of me, but I will not allow anyone to swear at me, and stay in their house. Her dad apologised to me and said it was just everything she has to deal with. I said that I understand that, and if they don't mind her swearing at them, that's fine, it's not my business, but I don't have to be spoken to in that way. If I am spoken to like that, I will not stay. Since then, she always glares at me, but she never swears at me. I hear her swearing at other people, and to her friends on the phone, but not at me.'

Whilst families should be allowed to choose how they live their lives and manage their relationships, you may be unable to be involved in some activities or practices because of legal constraints or employment requirements. The distinction between judging others, rejecting or questioning their decision-making, and situations where you are constrained by the requirements of the law, your employer or your own values and beliefs should be made clear (Hewitt-Taylor 2007). One of Tom's carers explains:

'Tom and his mates sometimes smoke joints and drink up at the rec, and that's up to them, it's none of my business. He comes back and I know what he's been doing, because he's a bit stoned. That's up to him, but while I'm with him, I say that it is illegal and I can't be involved, even in watching. I don't care what he does when I'm not around, I don't care what he's agreed with his family; if I am supposedly looking after him, and he is only 16, then he doesn't do it, because it could fall on my head. Sometimes I will go and collect him from the rec, and if he has already been smoking and drinking, that's up to him, but as soon as I take hold of his chair, he needs to be not smoking or drinking, or else he stays there without me.'

Trust

A relationship in which there is respect between staff and families makes it more likely that trust will develop. The existence of trust, like respect, does not imply that you agree with the child or family on everything. It means that you know and respect their wishes, values and beliefs; that any limits to what you are able to do or participate in are acknowledged; and that any concerns or differences of opinion are dealt with openly. In Tom's case, the relationship with his carer is one of trust; they may not agree on all his actions, but there is clarity over what each person's position is, and the agreement that has been reached is adhered to.

Respecting confidentiality is an important part of respecting a person, and honouring the trust invested in you (Johnson 2006, Nursing and Midwifery Council 2008). Maintaining confidentiality means that you do not disclose any information about a child or their family without their explicit permission (Nursing and Midwifery Council 2008). By working in a family's home, you have access to information about every aspect of their life. This may include information about the child's health, but also knowledge of the family members' preferences, beliefs, values, activities, relationships, home circumstances, environment and finances. This should all be regarded as confidential, unless otherwise agreed. We all know what we want other people to know, and not know, about us. In some cases, we also know that sharing what may seem like innocent information could be very damaging to ourselves or others.

It is a good idea to be completely clear about who can and cannot be given any information about the child or family you work with. This applies not only to health-related information, but to other information gleaned in the course of working in the family's home. This sometimes means that you have to explain very clearly to children, parents, and other family, friends or acquaintances why you have to withhold trivial-seeming information. One of Amelie's carers describes how:

> 'Once, when we were in the pub, a friend of a friend asked me: "Where is it you work?" and I said: "With a family whose daughter needs overnight care." She asked: "Is that that little girl in year two at Jake's school?" I said: "Oh, you know, I can't say really." It was awkward, but I thought, she obviously knows the family, or of the family, and one thing leads to another and it's better to just say nothing. It means I have to be really careful about what I say though. Usual work talk isn't really an option. Even if I just say: "The girl I work with was really messing around tonight," that might get back to someone or be misinterpreted or something, so you have to be really careful.'

Personal and professional boundaries

The relationship that you develop with the children and families you work with can be very satisfying. However, working in their homes often brings you into very close and undiluted contact with them and their circumstances, and can create problems in terms of the boundaries required for effective working (Samwell 2005, Hewitt-Taylor 2007). Although establishing good working relationships with children and their families is important, so too is maintaining personal and professional boundaries (Nursing and Midwifery Council 2008). It is relatively easy to accidentally overstep boundaries and to find that things develop into a difficult situation.

Samwell (2005) describes how families may develop the wrong impression about the intended or desired level of involvement that staff have with them. For example, parents may perceive that you are their friend – because you seem to get on well, because of the information you exchange in casual conversation, because of the time you spend together, or your apparent shared concern about the child. However, you may see your involvement solely as a part of your job, and your conversation as necessary small talk (Samwell 2005). Equally, you may make the error of judgment and think that a family sees you as a friend when they do not. As Samwell (2005) identifies, one of the most difficult aspects of working in a home setting is communicating an interest in and commitment to the family, being attentive to the needs of the child and their family as people, and establishing trust, without overstepping professional boundaries. One of Aisha's carers explains:

> 'We have this rule that we are just there to look after Aisha, not her siblings. Of course if they are all playing together we chat to them, and play with them all, we're not unfriendly, but we can't take responsibility for them. I always got on OK with her mum, and she had been telling me how tough it was, and I guess I'd been sympathising, as you do. Then she said: "Is it OK if I just pop to the shop and get some food for tea? Can you keep an eye on the kids?" Well, I can't do that, because we aren't insured for that, and if Aisha went off and I also had the others ... so I had to say "no" and it was awkward because I think, with having chatted to her, and being sympathetic, and because I was playing with them all, she expected me to help out like a friend would, not act like a staff member who had employment rules to follow.'

If very close bonds do form between yourself and the family you work with, it can be difficult for everyone concerned if you move on, and for the staff who replace you (Samwell 2005). In addition, if you become too involved in a family's life, your private time and emotional energy may become absorbed by your work with them, to the detriment of other aspects of your life (Samwell 2005). Equally, if you try to become more involved than the family find helpful they may find this intrusive and claustrophobic, but feel unable to say anything for fear of offending you (Hewitt-Taylor 2007).

The level of everyday involvement that you inevitably have with a family with whom you work closely, and the workload that many families have to juggle, may make you want to solve their problems for them. However, it is important to avoid establishing a relationship that encourages families to be dependent on you, and your views, opinions, or solutions to problems (Samwell 2005). What is best for one person or family will not necessarily be best for another, and the role you should usually take on is to assist families in identifying their needs, priorities and preferences, and to help them find ways in which these might be achieved or met. The intention should be to enable children, young people and their families to develop autonomy, not dependence on individual staff. James's mother recalls:

> 'One girl who worked here was always telling me what I should do. Not with James's oxygen or feeds, but basically what I should think and decide and do with my life, my house, everything. I think she meant to be kind and helpful, but it was "You should do this", "You should do that" and then, "So, have you done that then?" and I felt I had to explain why I hadn't if I didn't want to, and it got a bit annoying. I was glad when she left.'

Your rights

Although you are employed to support a child and their family, you also have a right to health and well-being at work. Employers have a statutory duty, as set out in the Health and Safety at Work Act (HMSO 1974), to take reasonable care of their employees' health and safety whilst they are at work, and this duty includes employees who work in families' homes (Taylor and Donnelly 2006). Your right to health and safety at work includes being able to use safe moving and handling techniques and not being required to compromise your personal safety. Links to information on health and safety at work issues are listed in Box 4 (below).

Box 4: Information on health, safety and well-being at work

Health and Safety Executive
http://www.hse.gov.uk
Health and safety at work advice
http://www.nhs.uk/Tools/Pages/WorkplaceHealth.aspx?Tag=Health+and+safety+
Information on rights and responsibilities related to health and safety at work
http://www.direct.gov.uk/en/Employment/HealthAndSafetyAtWork/index.htm

However, although your employer has a duty to safeguard your health and safety, you also have a responsibility to: highlight any threats to this, any concerns that you have, request appropriate training (for example, related to moving and handling or to personal safety), and to document any risks that you are required to take and how you have sought to resolve these. An assessment of the potential risks in the work environment should be completed before anyone starts to work in a family's home, but things may change as time progresses, and your employer may not be aware of the minutiae of your day-to-day work, and any risks that have developed or have been overlooked, unless you inform them of these.

As well as your physical safety, your well-being at work is important, and this may mean clarifying how the practicalities of balancing the family's needs and your rights will be achieved. This may include issues such as how the family's right to quiet at night will be managed alongside your need to carry out your work and, if necessary, communicate with other team members (Farasat and Hewitt-Taylor 2007, Hewitt-Taylor 2007). It may also concern how your right to privacy, as well as the family's, will be upheld; you have may have little time alone and your emotions, habits and behaviours may be subject to constant scrutiny by the child and family. It is useful to have such agreements in place at an early stage, so that both parties are clear on exactly what has been agreed as being 'reasonable'.

Whilst families have a right to conduct their lives and relationships as they see fit, and as best suits their preferences and values, the emotional atmosphere that their personalities and relationships create can sometimes be problematic for those who work in their homes. If there is an atmosphere of discontent or conflict in the home, this may be difficult to work with. You may be called upon to take sides in family arguments, and this can place you in a difficult position, especially if it occurs on a regular basis. Families should be clear from the outset that you do not expect to have to be involved in this type of situation, and it is best to make sure that nothing that you say, even in apparently neutral general sympathy, can be perceived as 'taking sides' in family matters.

Summary

Working in the home setting can be very rewarding but it also presents some specific challenges, which it is advisable to be aware of. The child and family, whilst needing and usually appreciating the help you give them, are likely to have their privacy compromised by your presence, and feel that their lives are intruded on to some degree. There will probably need to be constant negotiation of both the major aspects of a care package and the minor, everyday, aspects of working in the family home. This includes establishing mutual respect, and also clarity over the limits and boundaries within which your work is to be carried out. Respecting the child and family, and acting in a trustworthy manner, does not mean that you have no rights yourself. It is important for you to be aware of and maintain your own rights, including your right to work in a safe environment, and to make clear that you expect the respect you give the family to be reciprocated.

Chapter 8

Working with parents

Working with children almost always means working closely with their parents. In fact, it may often seem as if you work more with a child's parents than with the child themselves. Although working with parents is a major part of working with children, it is a mistake to assume that it will always be easy to identify who a child's parents are, or who has parental responsibility for them. A lot of the time it will be, but if a decision is needed urgently, and no one has established who can make it, or if someone makes a decision or takes an action and you are not sure if they have the right to do so, it becomes problematic. You therefore need to be aware of the legal arrangements related to childcare that are relevant to the families you work with.

At the same time, provided the parental arrangements fall within an acceptable legal framework, you should respect and work with them in whatever way they choose to organise their child's care. When a child has a long-term health problem, their parents will probably have had many challenges to face. Not having been in their position, it is usually better not to judge the decisions and arrangements they have made.

Experience of parenting

Having a child who needs long-term respiratory support often makes the experience of parenting very different from what people expected, and from the experiences of other parents. Their initial experiences with their newborn baby may be different from those they had anticipated. For example, Amelie's parents did not expect to have anything other than a 'healthy baby', and when Amelie was born, they had no reason to doubt this. However, a couple of hours after she was born she went to sleep, and stopped breathing. Her parents then had to begin to adapt their expectations very abruptly, in an unfamiliar environment. Instead of being taken home a few hours after her birth, Amelie was transferred to the neonatal intensive care unit (NICU), and did not go home until she was six months old. James was born at 25 weeks' gestation. His parents lost the last 15 weeks of preparation for his arrival that they had been expecting to have. Instead, this time was spent in the NICU, and James spent the first nine months of his life in hospital.

For both Amelie's and James's parents, the activities and nurturing that they were expecting to experience with their newborn baby were dramatically changed. James was separated from his parents as soon as he was born, because he required immediate intensive care, and Amelie was taken from her parents to the NICU very soon after she was born. James's parents could not hold him initially, because he was too unstable. They had their first cuddle with him a week after he was born. Because Amelie stopped breathing as soon as she went to sleep, she was intubated with an endotracheal tube and ventilated whilst she was asleep, which made holding her more difficult than it would otherwise have been. Both sets of parents had to divide their time between children at home and their babies in hospital, which meant that they could never be with either child as much as they had expected, or would have liked, to be.

As well as having to accept that the length, intensity and nature of their contact with their babies would not be the same as it would have been in other situations, James's and Amelie's parents had to develop their relationships with them in a public environment. In the neonatal unit, almost every moment of their time with their babies was spent in the company of a member of staff. James's parents could not even cuddle him without a staff member being with them, because they needed help to get him out of the incubator, position him, and keep his ventilation, infusion and monitoring lines intact. His mother recalls:

> 'I had been planning to have my second cuddle with him, but then just as we were about to do it, another baby needed urgent attention, so it didn't happen. Of course we understood, the other baby was very, very sick, but ordinarily you just don't have to plan every cuddle with your baby, and rely on nurses being free. There was no spontaneity in our world.'

If a child requires support once they go home, their parents' relationship with them may have to continue to be developed in the presence of others. Even when a family does not need 24-hour assistance, frequent visits from professionals, or staff being present in their home at night, can mean that they do not spend the time they expected to spend alone with their child, establishing their own routines and norms. They may feel that their relationship with their child, and their parenting style, are open to observation and comments by others, which they would not otherwise experience.

In other cases, it becomes apparent over the first few months of a baby's life that they have additional health needs. This can mean that their parents' early relationship with their child involves living through months of uncertainty. During this time, their baby is not as they expected, but the reasons for this, and the long-term implications of their condition, are unclear. Aisha's parents first began to suspect that something was wrong when she was only a week old, but she did not have a definitive diagnosis for another six months. Her parents had expected to enjoy having a new family member, but their time was instead filled with anxiety and tension; she did not meet her early motor milestones, had considerable difficulty in feeding, and was very different from the way their two other children had been as babies. Aisha's father left the family when she was four months old. Although there were a number of reasons for his departure, Aisha's mother suspects that the difference in what he expected and the reality, and uncertainty over what the problem was, and what their future held, were contributory factors.

When an older child develops a long-term respiratory problem, their parents' expected or established relationship with them, and expectations of their joint future, are likely to change. This process may again start in an unfamiliar environment, with little or no privacy. Fateha was involved in a road traffic accident in which her father was killed, and her mother had to adjust to her husband's death and her daughter's changed life in the paediatric intensive care unit of a hospital over 30km from her home. She also had her son to care for and comfort. The rest of her family were not living in the UK, so she had to manage this largely alone. Her changed expectation of parenting continued at home, where the family had to relocate and learn to live their new lives, negotiating this unknown territory mainly in the presence of strangers, because Fateha required 24-hour care. Fateha's mother recalls that:

'I became a single parent, with two children, one of whom was not really the child I had known. She is the same Fateha in her head, but instead of being my number one helper, joking with me, and being the life and soul of the family, she needed everything doing for her. Her brother, of course, was trying to understand that he had lost his dad, and his sister really, and I was trying to field all that. I had carers with me all day and night, which I needed because I couldn't manage all that and Fateha's care on my own, but in another way I felt as if I had to sort everything out in front of an audience. Put on a brave face, because they wouldn't want to work with a person who was falling apart. Sometimes I felt like I had to almost justify to them what I did and why. They never asked me to; it was just what I felt.'

The relationship that parents have, or perceive themselves to have, with their other children can also be affected by having one child who needs long-term respiratory support. Aisha's mother explains that:

'I have three children, but Aisha needs constant physical care. Kyle is only five, and he has just started school, and needs me to unscramble some of that with him. Sarah is seven, and has ballet and swimming and things like that, and she should be able to do those things, and have me with her, but the physical care Aisha needs makes it hard to do that. It's rare that I can take Sarah to swimming or ballet. One of the other mums does it, so she still goes, but she doesn't have her mum there.'

Parents may also feel that they lack privacy to be with their other children, and their concerns about the effect of one child's needs on the others can add to their stress (Taylor *et al*. 2001, Abbott *et al*. 2005). Fateha's mother recalls: 'One day Farid came in really upset, and I was hugging him, and one of the carers walked in, and he leapt up and left the room. He felt he was too big to be cuddling his mum, or to be seen doing it.'

Changed parenting roles

Parents whose children have additional health needs often develop a very special, intuitive and intensive knowledge of their child. Whilst this makes them uniquely able to meet their children's needs, it can also contribute to making parenting very different for them than it is for other parents, and can change their expected role as parents (Kirk *et al*. 2005). For example, if a baby cannot feed, or finds feeding difficult, what some people consider to be a very significant part of parenting may be lost, or become a source of struggle rather than an opportunity for developing a close relationship with their baby. Aisha had great difficulty in feeding, and her mother found this a tiring and frustrating, rather than enjoyable, time with her newborn baby. She describes how:

'With the other two, you snuggled up with them in the chair and, as they fed, they dozed off, and became soft and cuddly. With Aisha, it was one gulp, and she'd choke or vomit, and she was so floppy she could hardly latch on, because we couldn't get her in the right position, and we didn't know why. Feeding, which was one of my best times with the other two, was a nightmare.'

If a child requires assisted feeding, one of their parents' expected nurturing roles may become more like a clinical procedure than an intimate element of bonding with their child (Hazel 2006). James's mother had planned to breast-feed him, but, although she used expressed milk, he was tube fed for his first months of life. As she recalls: 'It's not quite the same ... being attached to a pump and then putting your milk down a tube...'

Parents whose children have additional health needs often have to perform procedures that are painful, uncomfortable or distressing, which runs counter to their expected role of protecting their children from suffering (Abbott *et al*. 2005, Kirk *et al*. 2005). This may include performing airway suction, changing tracheostomy tubes, or making their child keep an uncomfortable mask on. Parents are often specialists in their child's condition, and can sometimes appear to have a role that is more like that of a healthcare professional than a parent. However, whilst their specialist knowledge and skills should be recognised and valued, it is also important to remember that parents are primarily their child's parents, not healthcare providers. Their attachment to their child, and their feelings for them, are those of a parent, not those of a caring, but detached, professional (Kirk et al. 2005).

Working with expert parents

Parents whose children require long-term respiratory support are usually experts in their technical and healthcare requirements. They have unique knowledge of their child's condition; how their child responds to a range of situations and interventions; and, perhaps most importantly, they know their child as a person and how their health needs can be managed in the context of the family as a whole (Kirk et al. 2005, Hewitt-Taylor 2007). They are also usually able to detect changes in their child's state of health earlier than professionals can (Judson 2004, Kirk et al. 2005, Hewitt-Taylor 2007). However, some parents feel that professionals find their knowledge threatening, and that their expertise, especially where this is based on intuitive knowledge rather than objective, scientific, fact, is not always fully acknowledged (Kirk and Glendinning 2004, Kirk et al. 2005). Tom's father explains:

'We've got to know exactly what the signs of Tom being a bit under par are. Usually nothing medical: a bit grumpier, a bit less upbeat, and next day he has a chest infection. But "a bit grumpy" isn't a medical diagnosis, so people don't tend to act on that. But you do wonder, if they did, would it mean we got on top of things more quickly?'

Over time, parents whose children need long-term respiratory support may become adept at tweaking their treatment or interventions to meet their needs. They can often anticipate their child's condition changing, or are aware that a timely but slight alteration in what is being done is important. Whilst you may respect this, and their expertise, it can be difficult if they request that you make such changes when these are outside your remit. It is important to establish, alongside other boundaries, exactly what you can and cannot do, in terms of altering treatment or interventions; why this is; and where your responsibilities lie. It may be useful to clarify that, whilst you respect parents' right to manage their child's care as they see fit, you are obliged, legally, to follow the policies, protocols or guidance given by your employer. It is also sensible to know whom you can refer to if this becomes difficult. One of James's carers recounts this type of incident:

'His mum changes things a bit as she sees fit, but we have to follow the prescriptions and care plan we have. One night I came to work and she said "I've put his oxygen up by a quarter, and it can go up to 1.5 litres per minute if you think he needs it." Well, it's OK for her to do that, but our prescription says 1 litre per minute, so I had to say "OK, I'll just call the Team Leader and let her know." His mum made a kind of face, but I was looking after him all night, so if something happened and there I was giving him more than was prescribed, it could have been difficult for me. There was no problem. The Team Leader said "Fine, just document it" and she talked to James's mum and said that I wasn't allowed to put it up to 1.5, and she sighed and said "OK, call me then if you need to." I can understand how she felt, because it does seem petty and she needs her sleep, but that's the difference between it being up to her because he's her child, and it not being up to me, because I am employed to follow the care plan and prescription.'

At the same time, some parents have pointed out that, whilst they are the experts in their own children's care needs, they are not medically trained and they look to professionals to help them when they reach the limits of their knowledge. This includes occasions when new situations arise, or procedures or care that they are unfamiliar with become necessary (Hewitt-Taylor 2007). James's mother recalls one occasion when he had bronchiolitis:

'His everyday care, and his oxygen and tube feeding, I would say I am pretty much on top of things, and not much fazes me. The problem is, when he had bronchiolitis, everyone was assuming: "Well, it's still oxygen, and tube feeding, she's OK, she knows about it, we can leave her to it," but I wasn't OK, because the situation I was giving oxygen and feeds in was different, so I needed help just like any other parent would.'

Parents may also feel that they are relied upon to pass messages between professionals, or to teach them. This may not always be a problem, and it can be important for parents to see that professionals value them and are prepared to learn from them. However, at times it can place a burden of responsibility on the parents that they would rather not have (Miller *et al.* 2009). One of the challenges you face is to find a way of working in partnership with parents, sharing and valuing the knowledge, skills and resources they contribute, but without adding to their burden (Donaldson 2003). James's mother recalls:

'One time, when we had a new carer starting, the Team Leader said to me: "We have a new nurse starting, and we need to teach her all about James's care. We know that you know the most about it, but we don't want you to feel put upon, so if you'd like to help with her teaching, that would be great, but if you don't want to be involved, because it is our job to teach her, not yours, then that's fine too." I really appreciated that. It made me feel like they acknowledged me, but didn't want to dump on me. I sat down with her and we talked about what the new nurse would get taught and what it would be useful for me to be involved in or not, and what suited me, and it was really good. I felt really good about that.'

Workload

The level of care that some children need means that their parents are subject to considerable and ongoing physical demands and time management challenges (Heaton *et al.* 2005, Levine 2005). This includes the physical work of moving and handling their child and any equipment that they use, and assisting their child with eating, washing, dressing and toileting (Wang and Barnard 2004, Shribman 2007). Fateha requires all her physical needs to be met for her, and if she did not have carers, this would occupy almost all of her mother's time.

Although James's physical needs are less severe than Fateha's, even taking him on the short trip to his sisters' school is demanding for his mother. She recalls:

'The worst time was when Alice was in Reception class, because you had to take them right to the classroom door. So it was a case of getting James and his oxygen to the car, getting him and his oxygen in, putting his buggy in the boot, making sure Alice was in and had all her school things, getting them all out again at the school, getting Alice into class, then James plus oxygen plus buggy back to the car, and then out again at home. Now, if I can park near enough to the school, I can watch Alice run in, but if there's no parking nearby I still have to get James in and out each time. Parking near the school is a nightmare. There's no disabled parking, and I have to be able to get James and his equipment and chair in and out. That is pretty difficult if there are children and their parents trying to get past on the pavement and no space at the back to open the boot and get the chair out because everyone has to park so close. I have asked the school about disabled parking, but because he isn't a pupil they can't do anything, apparently. Luckily, his epilepsy is pretty well controlled, but if he does happen to have a seizure during that process, you really are thrown. At one point he did go through a phase of having more seizures, and I used to get ready at least 15 minutes early, because I was worried about Alice being late to school if we got held up.'

Many parents also spend a great deal of time arranging services for their child. James's mother explains that organising supplies of oxygen tubing, nasal prongs, transport oxygen and pulse oximetry probes, ordering prescriptions, making appointments, and discussing carer issues with the home care Team Leader, can take a long time. Parents may also experience long-term sleep deprivation because they need to attend to their child during the night, or because of the noise of machinery or alarms at night, which may be disruptive even when another person is employed to care for their child (Wang and Barnard 2004). James has a carer five nights a week, so his mother always has two nights when she has to sleep 'next to him, with one ear open', and then care for both her children during the day. She recalls:

> 'Sometimes, people acted as if I was asking for a luxury, asking for the night care, but you try looking after two under-fives, one of whom has additional needs, when you've had no sleep. Two days of no sleep is still too much.'

Some parents whose children require long-term respiratory support feel that they have no time 'off duty' from the physical care and vigilant watching that their child needs (Abbott et al. 2005, Kirk et al. 2005). Even when they are provided with assistance, or if their child ostensibly does not need constant care, they often still have to remain constantly available at short notice. Patryc's mother had considered going back to work when he started school, but has found this impossible because of the number of calls she still has to field, and all the times she has to go into school to show staff how things work, explain what Patryc can and cannot be involved in, and allay their concerns. In his first half term, there was only one day when she did not get a call, and she had to go into the school on 20 occasions for something related to his tracheostomy.

A child with long-term respiratory needs often requires a high level of care for much longer than would be the case for another child (Kirk and Glendinning 2004). In addition, as they grow older, their needs may become more demanding for their parents, because they become physically heavier or their condition deteriorates. When Tom was seven, he could walk, get himself in and out of the bath, and use the toilet unaided. He now uses a wheelchair, can only take one or two steps with a frame, needs to be lifted into the bath using a hoist, requires assistance to dry and dress himself, and uses a frame to transfer to the toilet.

Managing society's responses

As well as the physical demands and time management challenges that their child's care needs create, parents whose children need long-term respiratory support often have to contend with society's perceptions of, and reactions to, their child. Parents have reported hearing hurtful and dismissive comments about their babies and children, and, instead of a celebration of their lives and achievements, being asked about the likelihood of their survival and the possible value of their lives (Green 2002, Kirk and Glendinning 2004, Carnevale et al. 2006, Hewitt-Taylor 2007). Fateha's mother has overheard professionals and acquaintances discussing whether Fateha would have been better off being killed in the crash she was involved in.

James's mother reports hearing people say things like: 'You do wonder if they should just be left to die, when they're like that.' She explains: 'When I hear that, I think: "That's my son you're talking about! You should see the fun he has. How much he loves his trains, how he laughs and enjoys his life."'

Parents may not only have to hear such comments, but to develop ways of protecting their child from them, and helping them to learn to deal with them (Landsman 1998: 78). This can be emotionally draining, and may discourage them from going out with their children. Patryc's mother describes how every time they go out, someone will ask her about Patryc's tracheostomy. Not necessarily unkindly, but: 'They look at him, and see a sweet blond-haired little boy, and then they see the trache, and their faces change, and instead of saying "Hello, how old are you?" they say "What's that?" or "What happened" or "What a shame."'

Changes in social life and leisure activities

Parents whose children need long-term respiratory support may find it difficult to maintain friendships and contact with their peers because meeting their child's care needs, attending appointments, and organising services may leave them little or no time for this, or may make their schedules incompatible with those of their friends (Yantzi et al. 2006). If parents need to take their child with them to meet friends, the processes involved in this can make socialising more of a burden than a pleasure.

James's mother describes how:

> 'James used to be tube fed, or part tube fed, and I had to take everything I needed for that when we went out, but in some respects that was easy. Now he isn't tube fed, but he is really slow at eating, there's a limit to what he can eat, and he needs help because of his co-ordination, so you can't just meet a friend for lunch because lunch needs concentration by him and me. So that leaves the rest of the day. By the time we've got back from dropping Alice at school, and got him washed and dressed, because there is never time for him to have breakfast and get washed and dressed before we take Alice to school, it's almost ten o'clock, and he needs his snack. Then by that time, if I'm aiming to be back here for lunch, I haven't really got time to get James in the car again, and see anyone. After lunch, by the time he's finished eating, and I've cleared up, it's almost time to get him in the car to collect Alice. His meals take at least an hour, because he just can't eat faster. So, when you add those up, and the fact that he can't just run out to the car and get in, then really you have no time at all. When he was tube fed and Alice wasn't at school, I could go out more. So usually now I get my friends to come here, but you can't just expect everyone else to always do the running.'

Some parents are left so exhausted by meeting their child's needs that they simply do not have the energy to make plans to meet friends or family (Yantzi et al. 2006). James's mother comments:

'Someone once said to me: "Well, if he finishes lunch at one, then you could be out by half one, have an hour or so with a friend, and then pick Alice up." I suppose I could, and occasionally I do, but it's just the energy it takes. Actually I need that one hour in the day when nothing is happening except maybe me reading to James, or playing, or something. Not rushing out again or rushing lunch or feeling under pressure.'

As well as the practical considerations that may make it hard for parents to maintain friendships, when their child has additional needs they may feel that they no longer have a great deal in common with the people they used to socialise with. In some cases, their friends' reactions to their child, and failure to understand the demands and rewards of their role, may make it difficult for them to sustain existing friendships. Aisha's mother has found that, although she maintains contact with other parents because of her two older children: 'They do live in a different world from me, I don't feel I have much in common with them any more.'

Changes in employment and financial status

Having a child who needs long-term respiratory support often alters parents' employment opportunities. Mothers of disabled children are much less likely to be in paid employment than other mothers: 16% of mothers with disabled children are employed, compared with 61% of other mothers (Department of Health 2004a). Although many parents would welcome the opportunity to be involved in paid employment or activities that do not centre on their child's needs, this is often very difficult for them to achieve (Donovan et al. 2005, Judson 2004). Finding reliable care options for their child whilst they are at work is often almost impossible. Pre-school provision for children with additional health needs is often much more difficult to find than it is for other children, and, once a child is at school, finding suitable care for them during school holidays and after school can be difficult. James's mother explains:

'When Alice was three, she went to pre-school two days a week, and I did some part-time work at the library. But the pre-school attached to Alice's school, where she went, can't take James, because they can't manage his oxygen. There is one pre-school that can take him, but it's half an hour's drive away, so by the time I got him there, after dropping Alice off, it would be half past nine at the earliest. They said they couldn't manage him needing a longer lunch and help with feeding, so he couldn't do whole days. He could do the morning, which would be half nine by the time I got him there, to quarter to twelve, but by the time I had dropped him off and then got anywhere and then got back, that would give me about an hour and a quarter at the most to offer an employer. So, for me, work won't be an option until he gets into full-time school. If then.'

Parents often find that, even when their child is at school, they need to take time off work for hospital visits and appointments, and may also be unable to attend work more frequently than other parents, because their child is unwell, or if the school is unable to manage their child's needs (Contact a Family 2004b). Patryc's mother explains that when Patryc has a cough or cold (which, for any other child, would mean they came to school as normal) he cannot attend school:

> 'In Reception, they are all, always, full of colds and coughs, and that means that it seems as if Patryc never goes to school. I sent him in one day because he just had a cold, he hadn't got a temperature, he was fine, running around, coughing and sneezing but OK, but because he sounds different from the other children, and they were worried about his trache, they called me to bring him home. That happened five times, so now I just keep him off. He is not actually any iller than the other children, but he misses a lot more school.'

These things all mean that gaining and sustaining employment may be more difficult for parents whose children need long-term respiratory support than it is for other parents.

Changes in one or both parents' employment often have a major financial impact on families. Parents may receive state benefits because of their role in their child's care, but these rarely compensate for their salary losses (Abbott et al. 2005). In addition, the benefits to which parents are entitled are not always easy to find out about or claim (Department of Health 2004a, Abbot et al. 2005). Aisha's mother was a head teacher before Aisha was born, and, although she now receives state benefits, this is not equivalent to her previous salary and does not include the longer-term provision that her salary did, such as a pension. Aisha's father is an accountant and, since they have separated, their financial status is very different from what it was before.

At the same time as parents' income being reduced, the cost of housing adaptations, specialist furniture, toys their child can use, and incidental expenses such as transport and electricity mean that parents of disabled children often have higher outgoings than other parents (Department of Health 2004a, Hewitt-Taylor 2007). For example, Aisha cannot use many hand-me-down toys from her older siblings because they are mostly too bulky or heavy for her, and she cannot use the pushchair that her sisters used, because she needs a specially adapted buggy, which was expensive. Because she cannot go on outings with her other children very often, Aisha's mother spends more money on making sure that they can go out with their friends' families. They also have a CPAP machine running at night, and an oxygen concentrator during the day, both of which use additional electricity.

Overall, parents whose children have additional needs therefore often have more financial concerns than other parents. These parents have little control over these pressures, which can contribute significantly to their level of stress.

Changes in self-image

Changes to parents' employment may impact on their sense of self, as well as their financial stability. Going out to work can mean that they have a sense of identity other than as their child's parent. Although not all parents may want this, to many it is important (Todd and Jones 2005). Aisha's mother explains:

> 'I was a head teacher, and I enjoyed my work. I was part time, and in a job share, and we had organised for that to continue after a year's maternity leave, but now I have had to let that go. Sometimes I feel I am no one now, often I don't even have a name. I am "Aisha's mum". Much as I love my children, and love being their mum, sometimes it would be nice to be me as well.'

If parents can no longer work, it means they no longer have the opportunity to experience social interaction at work. Aisha's mother describes how:

> 'I used to see other people at work, and chat to them, but now I have mostly lost contact with them. So, I don't have that circle of friends or peers to talk to. It's not just the money: you do lose who you were. People used to see me and ask about work, and the girls, and Sean… Now they see me and just ask about Aisha. It's nice that they care, but people assume that all I can do or talk about is gastrostomy feeds and oxygen.'

For some parents, going out to work can act as a break from the demands of meeting their child's needs, and a lack of paid employment means that they do not have this opportunity (Yantzi et al. 2006). James's mother recalls: 'When I used to go to the library to work, I wouldn't say I loved my work, but it was a change, something different, where we had a laugh and adult conversation about something other than children. I don't get that now.'

Relationships between parents

Having a child who has additional health needs can bring couples closer together, but the pressures of looking after the child, organising their support, and having staff in their home can also place a strain on relationships (Contact a Family 2004a). James's mother describes how:

> 'Harry just couldn't take it, the whole oxygen and gastrostomy thing. He just found it too much. He said he just couldn't handle the care James needs, the long haul, so he left.'

Parents whose children need long-term respiratory support may find it difficult to enjoy time together and the usual range of babysitters, such as family and friends, cannot always manage their child's needs (Kirk and Glendinning 2004). Amelie's mother explains:

'You would think that it wasn't a big deal because Amelie only needs night care, but it can be. We were invited to an afternoon event, and I asked Mum if she could look after the girls, after lunch till about five, and she did, but she was worried in case Amelie fell asleep. She wouldn't let her lie on the sofa and watch TV, in case she dozed off.'

When parents have regular assistance with their child's care, it may mean that they have more time to be together, but having care staff present in the family home can also mean that they have very little privacy. When James's parents were in the process of separating, the only time they had to talk in private was after the carer arrived, and once Alice was also in bed. Although the carer being there gave them some time together, they were aware that what they said might be overheard, which constrained their conversation.

The role that each parent takes on in relation to their child and their needs may differ, and the effects of the child's needs may be very different for each partner. Amelie's mother and father had both planned to return to work, but her mother ended up leaving work to care for Amelie. She remembers how:

'We had decided that we would both work, and share childcare. But then, when it became clear that Amelie would be in hospital a long time, and then that we couldn't send her to nursery, we had to rethink, and I ended up not working again until last year. It was a decision we had to make, but it has meant that, career wise, I was disadvantaged, and I still am, because of that decision. It is always me that has to take time off for holidays or if they are ill. We were going to manage childcare equally, but the reality is that now it all falls on me. Even making their lunches, anything, it's me. That isn't what we had agreed when we decided to have another child. We used to come home and both talk about work, but then it was like, he had work to talk about and I had the girls, and we lost that common ground of moaning about work and we didn't both have work as a part of who we were; we started to have very different worlds. We lost the common ground we had planned to maintain, and we have never really got that back. Our jobs were kind of equal, but now my job is definitely seen as secondary, not just by Nigel, by everyone. They ask him about work, and ask me about the girls.'

The exhaustion that many parents experience may also be detrimental to relationships, as may stress over the organisational aspects of their child's care, and financial concerns (Hewitt-Taylor 2007). Parents may also have different views on their child's needs, respond differently to these, have different beliefs about how they should be catered for, and different ways of coping with the demands created by their child's needs (Hewitt-Taylor 2007). These may all create tension between partners, especially when their privacy and opportunities for uninterrupted discussion are limited.

Living with uncertainty

Many parents whose children have long-term respiratory problems have to live with almost constant uncertainty (Levine 2005, Meehan 2005), especially over their child's health (Buelow et al. 2006, Wang and Barnard 2004), and awareness of the frailty of their child's life (Redmond and Richardson 2003, Judson 2004, Carnevale et al. 2006). They also have to cope with uncertainty in the short term, every day, over how their child will be, and what they and their family will be able to do because of their child's needs. This often means that they learn to live and plan day to day, and that their outlook on life is very different from other people's (Redmond and Richardson 2003). Tom's mother explains:

> 'Ever since [Tom's brother] Adam was diagnosed, at five, we have tried to live a day at a time, whilst also having long-term plans. Trying to have plans for the future, so we didn't give up, and for Katie, because she has a future, but knowing that there is no long term for the boys. So we do focus on today a lot.'

Aisha's mother describes how:

> 'On the one hand, we know that we haven't got Aisha for long, so Kyle and Sarah and I want to spend our time with her, enjoying her. But they do have their own lives too, probably long lives. If Sarah misses out on swimming or ballet now, because of Aisha, then when will she catch up? So juggling what you really need to enjoy for the moment, because you may only have the moment, but also being fair to everyone, is hard. Often the bottom line is outside your control anyway because the final thing is: Aisha needs care and no one else is giving it, so that's me and I have to juggle everything around that anyway, regardless of the soul searching over what is right and fair. Sometimes I can't see beyond tomorrow, however much I should for the sake of the others, because today is just too demanding.'

The way parents view their situation may sometimes seem to be at odds with yours. One reason for this may be that, as well as having a different set of values and priorities, and knowing and valuing their child in a way that an outsider cannot always achieve, they are working in a different timeframe, which has to include a lot of people's needs.

Enabling parents to access support

The practicalities of caring for a child who requires long-term respiratory support can be exhausting and isolating for their parents. Whilst the day-to-day practical help that you provide may ease their physical burden, support organisations may assist them in other ways, and you may be well placed to suggest some of these organisations. Opportunities to meet, either face to face or via website forums, with people in similar situations may be useful in lessening their sense of isolation and stigmatisation, and creating a feeling of being understood and belonging. Such contacts may also enable parents to share ideas and strategies, and to give, as well as receive, support and assistance (Davies and Hall 2005). Box 3 (see page 74) shows some online peer support networks which parents may find useful, and Box 5 (below) shows some other sources of information and support for carers, and families of disabled children, which parents may find helpful.

Box 5: Sources of information and support for parents

Carers UK: an organisation that provides carers with information and advice
http://www.carersuk.org

Contact a Family: A UK-wide charity providing support, advice and information for families of disabled children
http://www.cafamily.org.uk/

Crossroads: Caring for Carers: an organisation that provides practical support for carers
http://www.crossroads.org.uk

Parents for Inclusion: a network of parents who promote the inclusion of children with disabilities and special needs in all areas of life
http://www.parentsforinclusion.org

Special Needs Kids: an information source for parents and carers
http://www.special-needs-kids.co.uk/index.htm

The Princess Royal Trust for Carers: a Trust that provides information, advice and support for carers (including young carers)
http://www.carers.org/

UK Government website: information for parents of disabled children
http://www.direct.gov.uk/en/CaringForSomeone/CaringForADisabledChild/index.htm

Many parents are unaware of, or fail to claim, the state benefits to which they are entitled, or to apply for funds that might be available to them (Department of Health 2004a, Hewitt-Taylor

2007). You may not be aware of all the benefits or allowances to which parents may be entitled, or their rights at work, but you may be in a position to suggest agencies or individuals who might provide them with information or assistance in this respect. Such recommendations or suggestions may also help parents to feel more comfortable about claiming their entitlements. James's mother recalls how:

> 'One nurse said to me: "Did you think of claiming for electricity? I think you can." She didn't actually know the process, but the idea put me onto it, and her suggesting it meant I felt less of a scrounger. It does take a fair bit of electricity, running a sats monitor, and an oxygen concentrator, and at one stage a feed pump too, overnight.'

As well as recommending and referring families to services or facilities, you should be aware of the reasons why they may not seek, or be reluctant to seek or accept, such support. Some families may prefer to manage alone, and perhaps find extra support or advice intrusive. In addition, some parents may see asking for support as an admission of failure, or letting their child down because it somehow implies that they are a burden, rather than a child who is loved and valued. A part of showing the value that they attach to their child can be caring for them (Brett 2004). Acknowledging the complexity of factors that influence what support parents find useful is a key part of providing them with a level and type of assistance that they will appreciate and find helpful.

Rewards

Although, for many parents whose children have additional needs, the long-term nature of their responsibility is demanding and exhausting, it can also be very rewarding. Most of the stress they experience is due to the practicalities of the care their child needs, the organisational factors they have to contend with, the social barriers they encounter, and the stigma that society creates, not the child themselves (Green 2007). Parents have described the love and hope they experience with their child (Kearney and Griffin 2001), and the value of their child's positive attributes, personal qualities, and lives (Landsman 2005). The child's presence may enable their parents to develop qualities such as tolerance and develop new values, priorities and beliefs (Scorgie and Sobsey 2000, Green 2002, Wolfson 2004, Lassetter et al. 2007). Nevertheless, these positive aspects of their relationship with their child and caring for them may be misinterpreted or devalued by others (Todd and Jones 2005). Aisha's mother comments:

> 'One of the women I worked with came to visit once, and I said something about, well at least I'm learning something new every day: feeds, CPAP and all that. But I also said that it is amazing how Aisha, who really can't do much, has the ability to make us all laugh,

and teaches me to be patient and think about every aspect of a situation, and enjoy the moment. Then I heard she told some other people at work: "I suppose she has to think that..." but I don't have to think it. It is actually true.'

Summary

Working with parents is an integral part of caring for children who require long-term respiratory support. Parents should all be seen as individuals, with no assumptions made about what they may feel, or what their circumstances may be. Nevertheless, it can be useful to have some awareness of how their anticipated role as parents may have changed because of their child's needs, and the changed roles, workload and lifestyle that they and their family may have, as a result. It is also worth considering how their new life with their child may have changed their relationships with others, and the way they see themselves and society. Whilst respecting and valuing parents' expertise in caring for their child, it is also important for you to provide them with adequate support and assistance. It can also be very useful to clarify how and why your role and allowable level of decision-making may differ from theirs, so that differences between their roles and responsibilities and yours can be understood and managed.

Chapter 9

Working with the whole family

Having a child who needs long-term respiratory support may change not only their parents' lives and experiences of parenting, but also the lives of the whole family. This can include their siblings, grandparents, aunts, uncles, and anyone else who is close to the child and their parents.

Whilst having staff to assist with a child's day-to-day care may give the parents time to spend with other family members, it can also mean that the family's life is conducted alongside comparative strangers, and that they feel that their interactions, emotions, behaviour and lifestyle are open to public inspection and judgment (Brett 2004, Kirk et al. 2005). Fateha's mother explains:

'I am lucky in that I have carers here almost constantly, which means I can spend some time with Farid. But having time completely alone with him can be a problem. At weekends, if he is not doing anything with his mates, I sometimes like to find a way for us to go out together for a while, because then there is just us. If not, nice though it is to have a family outing, and, although the carers are great, he has to talk to me with other people around, and he doesn't always want to do that. Even small things, like asking how school was, if he's done well, or not so well, he doesn't want someone else to be the first to hear. The other week he was trying out for the rugby team, and when he got in from school I was desperate to know how he'd got on, but the carer was there, so I had to say "Hi", and then "How's things?" He looked at me and had this big grin, so I knew he understood and had been chosen. But if he hadn't, or didn't want to say, I was trying to make it OK for him, in front of the carer, but also to make sure he knew I had remembered and was desperate to know.'

The family home

Whilst living in suitable housing and having appropriate equipment and assistive technology are necessary to enable a child or young person's health needs to be met, they can also alter the family's home beyond recognition. For example, finding space to store equipment and supplies can be difficult, and the family home may need to be adapted to accommodate a child's mobility problems or the assistive technology that they need. James's mother explains that they had planned for him to share a room with his sister until he was about five:

> 'But when you've got feeds, a saturation monitor and an oxygen concentrator going all night, you can't do that. So, his dad and I moved into the box room, which just about fits a double bed in, and he had our room. Then there was storage, of everything that used to be in the box room, and the equipment that James needs, of which you get a month's supply at a time. That was one of the things that his dad just couldn't hack – the clutter, as he called it. I still sleep in the box room, and what was our dining room has become the store room. It's OK, but it means we don't have much space, and we can't have visitors. We probably wouldn't anyway, but one time my sister said: "I'll come and stay and help you" and I thought "Where would I put her?"'

In some cases, families have to relocate to a more suitable property (Abbott et al. 2005). Whilst this may be essential, it disrupts their situation and can mean that their house is no longer the home they chose, or wanted (Hewitt-Taylor 2007). Fateha's mother has moved to a property that has a downstairs bedroom for Fateha. Whilst this was a necessary move, she explains that: 'We had to move because we couldn't manage in the other house. It was big enough, but impractical, because it couldn't take a stair lift and it had no downstairs facilities. But for Farid, it meant that he moved away from his friends, at a time when he really needed some stability. He had had his room decorated six weeks before the accident, exactly as he wanted it. It broke his heart to leave that room. We tried to do his room here up the same, but it isn't the room he and his dad designed. He never complains, but I saw his face when we moved and I know he misses his room, and everything it meant, including the memories of him and his dad doing it up.'

Family outings

When a child needs long-term respiratory support, their needs, and the number of appointments that their parents have to take them to, can make family outings problematic (Kirk and Glendinning 2004, Wang and Barnard 2004, Abbott et al. 2005). Fateha's mother explains:

> 'We were trying to organise some family days out in the summer holidays: by the time we

ruled out days when Fateha had appointments, and meetings, and deliveries of supplies, there weren't that many days left. People sometimes assume that a disabled child has a very empty life. It's not as if she has a lot of fun, but the majority of inflexible things in our family diary are about Fateha.'

When parents can organise days out for the whole family, finding locations that everyone will enjoy can present immense challenges (Rehm and Bradley 2005). James's mother recalls one outing that they went on:

'James's sister, Alice, was desperate to go to this local theme park. All her friends were going, and she kept talking about it. I kept delaying and fobbing her off, because I knew it would be difficult, but eventually I decided we'd go. The parking was miles from the entrance, and I was wheeling James, with oxygen and spare oxygen and his other bits and pieces. Then James can't get on the rides, because we'd have to lug him and his oxygen on, and position him, and do something with the chair, because that has the spare oxygen and supplies on it. Most of the rides, in fact all of them, can't take a wheelchair. Alice is only five, so she needs supervision, and holding onto sometimes, and there was hardly anything she could go on alone. There was a little train we could all get on, because it took big buggies or wheelchairs. She did seem to enjoy it, but I told her dad that he has to take her on her own one weekend, so she can do everything she wants to, and not have to spend an hour watching James eat his lunch when she's wolfed hers in ten minutes and wants to go back to the park.'

Fateha's mother likes to take both her children on days out, but finding places to stop for a meal can present a challenge. Fateha is fed via a gastrostomy and whilst her eating is therefore not an issue, finding somewhere that can easily accommodate her chair and equipment can be difficult. Her mother explains:

'I wouldn't bother about finding somewhere to eat, because I can just take a sandwich, and some of the carers find it awkward, I know, because the agreement is that we buy for them too. I think that's only fair because they wouldn't eat out if it wasn't for being with us, but some of them find that uncomfortable, so it's not an easy situation. But Farid's friends have days out and have burger meals and all that, so why shouldn't he? Then sometimes I look at the carer feeling awkward, and Farid trying to enjoy himself for my sake, and me acting cheerful like this is a great day out, and I think: "Who am I trying to kid?" This isn't like the family days out his mates have.'

As Fateha gets older, it is also becoming more difficult to find places to change her on days out, because, although most disabled toilets are large enough for her chair, equipment and carer, if she needs to lie down to be changed, there are very few places where this can be achieved with comfort and dignity. Her mother comments:

> 'Changing Fateha on days out is becoming a real issue. It's OK if we can just transfer her onto the toilet, but if she needs changing, or cleaning, then you are a bit stuck, because almost nowhere has those facilities. At the moment I am carrying a fleecy blanket around, and we have to find a big enough disabled toilet and lie her on the floor on that if needs be. But getting her down onto that, and then back up again, without dislodging her ventilator, or injuring her or us, is becoming a big problem.'

Even when suitable venues can be found, days out that include a child who needs long-term respiratory support often have to end earlier than would usually be the case because the family need to be home in time for them to begin therapies, feeds, or for staff to arrive (Kirk and Glendinning 2004). Tom's father's comment illustrates this point:

> 'Tom is meant to have BiPAP from ten. No one actually minds if it's a bit later, and if we let the carers know he'll be out later than that, or if they arrive and have to wait, as long as someone's there to let them in so they're not on the doorstep they are fine about it. So it's not as if anyone enforces it, or insists, but you have to be aware of it and let someone know, out of courtesy, if things have changed. It's just another consideration that we have if we go out. The other day we'd been over to see his uncle, and we stopped for something to eat on the way home, and I had to call the carer to say we'd be late. It's not a big deal, but it is an extra thing we have to think about that other families don't.'

Holidays

Going on a family holiday with a child who requires respiratory support often means many months of planning and organisation. Finding accommodation that meets the child's needs, and those of the whole family, can be difficult. Amelie's family have to find holiday accommodation that has a bedroom with enough plug points and room for her ventilator. Because she needs the ventilator at night, she has to have a room of her own, rather than sharing with her sister, which increases the cost of the holiday. Because Amelie's carers can only work locally, the family has to decide whether one parent will stay awake each night, or whether to find and pay for carers at the locality. Her mother describes how: 'Usually I end up deciding to muddle through. I doze in her room at night, because unless there's an alarm she is OK, but it means I always come back from holiday exhausted.'

Families also have to transport all the equipment and supplies that their children will need during the holiday. James's mother recalls a holiday that they took when he was two:

'I thought, well, at least we can just use a regular cottage, because at the time I could still carry him easily, but then we had to pack the car with his equipment: adapted buggy, oxygen concentrator, oxygen cylinders, tubing for oxygen, spare prongs, nasogastric tubes, feeding sets, pump, feeds for the week, saturation monitor and probes, medications. That was before we started on the regular holiday kit. We needed a bigger car really, but to hire one was a problem because of the oxygen and insurance, so we somehow got everything into our car. Then when we got there I realised that the electricity was metered and you had to put 50 pences in. A sats monitor, feed pump and an oxygen concentrator eat it up, so we needed to spend all day collecting 50 pences. I went to the bank one day and asked for 50 pences, but because it wasn't my bank they said no, and there wasn't a branch of my bank in that town. It was our holiday game: collecting 50 pences.'

Fateha's family find it very difficult to go on holiday, mainly because of the problems involved in finding suitable accommodation. Fateha's mother explains all the aspects that need to be considered:

'We need accommodation with an extra room for the carers to sleep in, so that makes it four bedrooms. We also have to have a place that has ramps and that has a bathroom Fateha can use: if it has a bath or shower that isn't "walk in" then we need a hoist or special chair, which we'd have to take with us, and we need a toilet with rails, and that is big enough to get her, the ventilator, chair and transfer equipment into. We also need a bedroom that is big enough, with a bed that's the right height for the carer and me to transfer her. You also have to check that the place really is accessible. One place I looked at said it was accessible for disabled people, but looking at the pictures, the only bedroom that would be big enough for her and her equipment was down a couple of steps. There was an accessible bedroom, but it was too small, we'd never have been able to get her into bed there because of her chair not fitting in at a sensible angle so you could also keep her ventilator attached to the chair whilst transferring her. So it's a case of checking the fine detail and finding there is not that much available. We did find one holiday complex with suitable accommodation, so we went there twice, because it was somewhere we knew worked. But then you feel you are going on holiday for the sake of it, to prove you can, not because anyone actually wants to go there.'

When a child has siblings, their enjoyment of holidays also has to be considered, Fateha's mother comments:

'It's hard to find something suitable for Fateha, but to find something that is suitable for Fateha and which Farid will enjoy too is impossible really. Last year we found another place that catered for disabled people, and when we arrived I saw him looking at all the other people in wheelchairs, and I thought: "This isn't fair on him." I think that children of all abilities mixing is good, but I thought: "This isn't so much mixing, as Farid only getting to be with disabled kids. He needs to be with other kids as well, who can do what he can." So this year I made the decision to leave Fateha at home with the carers for a week and take Farid to Spain on my own. I have mixed feelings about it, because I believe in the family being together, but Farid has a right to enjoy himself too.'

Holiday insurance is usually much higher for children with additional health needs than it is for other children. And if a family with a child who needs long-term respiratory support plan to travel abroad, it may be so expensive that they cannot even consider it. Amelie's mother has looked into the family going to Canada, but health insurance for Amelie alone would be over £1000. Going abroad not only attracts high insurance, but means considering in-flight facilities, equipment needs and mobility issues. Fateha's mother explains:

'We just could not take Fateha abroad – even to a nearby place like Spain. The cost would be huge, but there are also the practicalities. We could get her on the plane OK, and get her into a seat: she'd need a head support, and a special seatbelt, but we could do it. She'd need the ventilator and trache equipment in-flight, and a spare ventilator in case that one packed up, and an ambu bag and suction equipment, and also probably feeding equipment, and monitoring equipment because, although she doesn't have sats monitoring all the time, you'd need it on a flight, with the pressure changes. Then we'd need medications, and letters to get those through customs, so that's quite a lot of hand luggage. That's just for her medical needs. Finding accommodation in another country and being sure it was OK would be difficult, and then there's getting from the airport to the place you're staying, because we'd need a large taxi that was happy to take all our things, and to wait while we got Fateha and her chair in and out. It gets too tiring for me to think of. That's just the planning and Fateha's needs for the journey, before the holiday even begins.'

Even when a child has a less constant need for respiratory support, the practicalities of travelling abroad can be difficult. For Amelie to go to Canada, as well as the cost involved, her family would need to take a ventilator to use on the aeroplane, because of the duration of the flight, and, as well as their regular luggage, would need supplies for the ventilator circuit during the holiday, a back-up ventilator in case one fails, and an ambu bag for emergency use. As her father notes:

'That's a lot of extra luggage to take. It means you have to hire a much bigger car, and make sure the plug adapters you take will be good enough to support a ventilator, because it's not as if you can afford for the plug to be a bit of a wobbly connection.'

This combination of factors means that for many families who have a child who requires respiratory support, holidays, even within the UK, are difficult, if not impossible, and exhausting, to arrange (Abbott *et al.* 2005).

Siblings

It can be very difficult for a child when their sibling has additional needs. Although they may have a good relationship with their brother or sister, recognising the challenges they may face as siblings is an important part of providing support for the family.

A child who has additional needs often requires extra attention, or needs more of their parents' time, making it hard for siblings to get their 'fair share', which can make their brother or sister feel resentful. However, at the same time, because they realise that their sibling has additional needs, they may feel guilty for having such thoughts. Aisha's mother reports how:

> 'My other daughter, who is only seven, asked me the other day if she could have a friend to sleep over, and she must have seen my face because she then said: "Oh it's OK." I could see she was disappointed, so I said: "Yes. It's no problem." She said: "I know I'm lucky, because I'm not ill like Aisha, but I would like a sleepover Mummy." That just about broke my heart, because she was trying to think of her sister and me, but she does still have her own needs, and they should be recognised.'

Children whose brother or sister needs respiratory assistance may have their sleep disrupted because they are woken by their sibling, are aware of others attending to them, or can hear the noise of machinery or staff. James's mother describes how:

> 'Alice has her room just near James's, and when he was first home, she had a terrible time trying to sleep, because the sats alarm would go off, and the oxygen concentrator is noisy, but what really bothered her was that she could see the flickering red numbers on the sats monitor. They scared her at night. So we had to make sure they were out of her view. I forgot she had a mirror on her wall, and she could see the reflection of it even when we moved it. On the nights when we have a carer, we can shut the door, but when it's me, I'm in his room and she has to be able to come and find me if she wakes up and needs anything. I can't leave James for long, so instead of me taking her back to her room and settling her, she ends up snuggling up with me some nights. By morning there we are in this three-bedroom house, with James asleep in his bed, surrounded by equipment, and Alice and I squashed up on the single sofa bed that I put beside his bed, neither of us getting much sleep.'

Lack of sleep can mean that children feel tired during the day, which may affect their concentration and performance at school, their ability to complete homework, and their inclination to join in activities with their peers. In the longer term, this may affect their life opportunities. They may also find it difficult to join in out-of-school activities because of their brother or sister's needs (McClure 2005, Carnevale *et al.* 2006, Contact a Family 2007, Kirk and Glendinning 2004). Aisha's mother's comment illustrates this point:

> 'The other day, Sarah said that her class were going to London for the day, and she wanted to go. But they had to be in school at eight o'clock on a Saturday, which would mean leaving here at half seven. The first thing I thought was: "How am I going to manage that?" We have overnight carers, but they finish at eight, and I wouldn't be back in time if I dropped Sarah off. The other option would be getting Aisha up and taking her as well, like I do to get the children to school, but because she takes a while to get up and sorted that would mean a very early start. Just as I was running those options through my mind, Sarah said: "It's OK, Mum, Nadine's mum can pick me up." She'd thought about it, and organised it, all I had to do was sign the form, and she's only seven. I'd love to drop her off, like a proper mum. We are lucky because they have friends, and other people will help out, but they never have their mum to do it.'

Having a sibling with additional needs may also alter their brother or sister's social opportunities because of financial issues, which reduce the money available for them. Amelie's mother explains:

> 'We are not too badly off financially, but we lost my salary for a while, and now it is lower than it would have been, and we moved to a bigger house. So our budget has changed, and there are things that I have to say "no" to, which before, and if Amelie hadn't had the needs she has, I would have said "yes" to. Nothing major, but our financial status has changed and that naturally has an impact on the girls and what they can do now, and also for the future. University fees, deposits for a house, everything. The available pot is less than it would have been.'

Siblings' social opportunities may also be affected by other changes in their family's circumstances. Fateha's family had to move house after her accident, and her brother's existing friendship group was broken up, and he had to make new friends. He used to enjoy inviting friends to his house after school and at weekends, but now finds it difficult to do so because of the way they respond to his sister, and because there are always carers there.

Sometimes, uncertainty over a child's needs means that their siblings cannot count on enjoying events that have been planned. James's mother describes how:

> 'Alice had her birthday and wanted a party. So I said yes, and we had it all planned. Then James got sick and needed to be in hospital. He was sick, but he wasn't that sick, and so

I left him there and came home and did the party, because she misses out so much. I thought: "He's in safe hands, and for once, it's going to be her day." So many times I have said "Yes, let's go to the park" or "maybe we can go to the beach" and then we can't, because of James's needs, or because he has a cough or cold or is just not quite well enough. We don't plan big trips much, but even the small things get cancelled. I can't even promise to do her reading with her because it depends a bit on whether James is brewing something and all grumpy and unsettled. I know the hospital staff were a bit sniffy about it, because they expect me to stay, but if you have two children, they both count, and that was one day when it was her big day and someone else could look after James.'

The siblings of children who look physically different from other children may be teased or bullied because of this, or hear unkind or derogatory remarks about their brother or sister. Even remarks that are not intended to be unkind may be difficult for them to deal with. Tom's mother recalls:

'His sister came back from school one day when she was about seven and said: "Why did Adam have his legs chopped off?" Someone at school had said he had, because he was using a wheelchair, and it really scared her.'

Children may also be embarrassed by their brother or sister's appearance, behaviour, or because of the way other people react to them (Contact a Family 2007). Fateha's brother does not attend the same school as her, and their mother is pleased about this. She explains:

'At school, Farid can just be himself. I am aware that when he brings his friends here, he does sort of have to take a deep breath and explain his sister. I know he tries not to bring his friends here unless he knows them really well, whereas before, we used to have his friends and classmates dropping by any time.'

The siblings of children who have additional health needs may feel that they have less of their parents' time or attention than they otherwise would. This may be because the focus is on the sick child, and the time taken for their care leaves little time for other things, or because their parents are themselves suffering loss and cannot focus very easily on their other children's needs. From the child's perspective though, they may feel that their parents, as well as their sibling, have changed or been lost, and that they no longer love them, or no longer love them as much as they once did (Saldinger et al. 1999). Tom's mother describes her feelings:

'My daughter only has a tiny bit of us, really, because we have had to do so much with Adam and Tom. I feel like she has to fend for herself, and one day, when they are both gone, we will look at her and realise that she is our only child and we don't know her. I try every day to stop that happening but I don't think I have managed it.'

Aisha's mother heard her daughter saying to her five-year-old brother: 'Mummy has to spend more time with Aisha now, because she is very poorly, and then when Aisha is in heaven, Mummy will come back to us.'

As well as consideration of their immediate situation, one child's needs may affect their brother's or sister's future plans. Fateha's mother says:

> 'I don't want Farid to think he will have to pick up Fateha's care. He is a good son and brother, but I don't want this to become his life. He has lost a father and sister, and I don't want him to lose his future. So I keep just dropping hints, even though he's young, mentioning in passing how the carers also care for adults and that Fateha will always have carers, so that he knows she is catered for. I worry what she will do when I am gone, but I don't want him to worry about that too.'

Children whose siblings have long-term respiratory needs may provide for some of their care needs, or take on additional responsibilities because of their needs. These can include: household tasks, shopping, physical care, providing emotional support to their sibling and other family members, caring for other siblings and interpreting (Dearden and Becker 2004). These responsibilities may affect a number of areas of their lives, including their education, leisure activities and peer relationships (McClure 2005). The Department of Health (2004b) have recognised that siblings' needs should be taken into account when designing care packages for disabled children. It may not be your role to provide care or supervision for the siblings of the child you work with, but if you notice that they are being disadvantaged, or have needs that are being left unmet because of their brother's or sister's needs, you may be well placed to highlight this. You may also be able to encourage and support families in seeking a good deal for all their children, not just those who need long-term respiratory support.

Being obliged, or feeling obliged, to put their brother's or sister's needs first can mean that the siblings of children who have long-term health needs are unusually mature for their age, and their parents often worry that they have to take on too much responsibility and have to grow up too quickly. However, siblings of disabled children are also often described as very responsible and sensitive to the needs and feelings of others (Contact a Family 2007, Hewitt-Taylor 2007). The effects of having a sibling with additional needs can vary a great deal, and it would be wrong to suggest that having a brother or sister who requires long-term respiratory support is a negative experience (Taylor et al. 2001, Sharpe and Rossiter 2002, Contact a Family 2007). However, being aware of the extra challenges that may exist for the siblings of the children you work with, and trying to help them and their families to reduce any disadvantage they might encounter, is important. It may also be useful to suggest support and information resources for siblings, such as those in listed in Box 6 (below), to the families with whom you work.

Box 6: Organisations for siblings

Sibs: a charity for people who grow up with a brother or sister with special needs, disability, or chronic illness
http://www.sibs.org.uk/

Young Carers Net: an organisation that provides information and support for young carers
http://www.youngcarers.net

Extended family

A child having additional health needs can affect their extended family and friends as well as their parents and siblings (Contact a Family 2005). The effect their needs have will depend on the family structure and functions, but grandparents are often affected (Green 2001). When a child is critically ill, their grandparents have been described as having concerns for the well-being of both their child and grandchild (Hall 2004). The same may apply to people whose grandchild needs long-term respiratory support. Aisha's grandmother worries about her daughter and her grandchildren, but the person she worries about least is Aisha. She says:

> 'I worry about my daughter, and her health, and that she has lost her job, everything she worked for, and that she has financial worries, through no fault of her own. I also worry about the other two. The things they miss out on, and that they no longer see their dad. I do feel sorry for and grieve for Aisha, but she is not my biggest worry. I can't get too involved in looking after her anyway, so I suppose I haven't formed that link with her, but I do spend a lot of time with the other two, and I grieve for them and their mother, and feel hurt for them.'

Grandparents, like parents, may have a very different role from that which they expected. James's grandmother had done a great deal of babysitting for Alice, but now that she cannot look after both children, her visits to the family are less frequent. She only really sees the children with their mother, and is not a useful babysitter, but a visitor, who has to be catered for, along with everything else her daughter juggles.

Grandparents may have to deal with other people's reactions to their grandchildren, including prejudice, negative attitudes, thoughtless comments and awkwardness in discussing them. Aisha's grandmother comments:

> 'Being Aisha's granny is completely different from being the other two's granny. I am always telling my neighbour what the other two are up to and showing them photos, but with Aisha, I don't have that conversation, because there is nothing to say. She is a lovely little girl, but other than asking if she has a chest infection, my neighbour doesn't know what to talk about with her, and neither do I really. It's: "Sarah is doing this, and Kyle is doing that, and up to whatever mischief at school, and then... Aisha is ... Aisha." And the conversation ends.'

If a child's parents separate, this can also make things very different for their grandparents. Aisha's mother describes how:

> 'The children used to get on really well with Sean's mum and dad, but now they hardly ever see them. I don't know if they want to come over, but I expect they'd feel awkward, because Sean never contacts us. They haven't seen Aisha since she was about a year old, and I don't have the time or inclination to contact them. But they are missing out on their grandchildren, not just Aisha, but the other two, and I think the children miss them as well.'

Other members of the extended family may also have to deal with changes in their expected role when a child needs long-term respiratory support. Patryc's aunt lives nearby and had planned to help with her sister's childcare and school runs, but, although she can manage Patryc's tracheostomy, she does not feel confident enough to go to the school to sort out any problems associated with it, so there are limits on what she can do to help her sister. Other members of the child's family may, like their parents and grandparents, have to manage other people's views and comments on the child and their parents, have a double concern for the child and their parents, and feel unsure of the best way to support them.

Summary

When a child needs long-term respiratory support it is likely to affect their whole family in one way or another. This includes their home being altered, family outings and holidays changing, and the whole family structure altering. Siblings may need special consideration, so that their needs (as well as those of their brother or sister) are met, and so that they too have time to spend with their parents. It may also be helpful to consider how the extended family and friends are affected by a child's additional needs.

Chapter 10

Working with young people who require long-term respiratory support

The increasing number of children who need long-term respiratory support, and the medical and technical developments that have increased their life expectancies, mean that there is a growing population of teenagers who have this type of need (Chamberlain and Kent 2005, Department for Education and Skills and Department of Health 2006). Although many of the needs that adolescents have are similar to those they had as children, they face some specific challenges as they reach young adulthood. If you work with a child or young person these are important considerations, as part of their current care, or planning for their future.

Self-image

Adolescence can be a time at which young people's self-image and self-concept are particularly important, and contribute to the development of their self-esteem. Developing a positive sense of self-esteem can be challenging for any young person, but when they need long-term respiratory support, it may be even more difficult than usual for them to achieve this (Strandmark 2004, Christie and Viner 2005). The popular media tend to present physical perfection as the ideal to aspire to, which means that those who cannot conform to this may perceive themselves as less acceptable than their peers (Breakey 1997). Amelie's mother describes how Amelie wants to:

'…look and act like her friends: she doesn't want to be different. In the daytime, she isn't any different, and she hates people knowing about the fact that she needs ventilation at night, because it means she is different. As she gets older, it is probably going to matter more and more. Once she starts wanting to go out at night, and having boyfriends, needing night-time ventilation is going to matter even more than it does now.'

Whilst you cannot directly alter media stereotypes, you may be in a position to assist the young people you work with to see and value their positive attributes, highlight positive role models for them, and help them to decide how to manage their needs and other people's attitudes towards them.

Developing independence

During adolescence, young people explore their personal values, refine their personal identity, and develop the skills they will need to function in adult relationships. As a part of this, they negotiate new relationships with their family, and develop a degree of emotional, personal and financial independence from their parents (Christie and Viner 2005, Turner 2006). These developments are equally important for young people who need long-term respiratory support, but they may have much greater difficulty in achieving them. This can be partly because other people confuse their physical needs with their ability to develop independence (Department for Education and Skills and Department of Health 2006). As Fateha's mother explains: 'Fateha will never be able to meet her own physical needs, but she knows what she wants, and I want her to be able to make as many choices as she can about her life. She is very independent minded, she always was, and she gets very frustrated because physically she can't be independent, and people treat her as if she can't think for herself, but she most certainly can!'

One part of developing independence is young people having the opportunity to explore their views, values and plans with their peers. However, if they need someone to be with them when they meet their peers, their opportunities to do this, and the conversations that they have when they do so, may be constrained, especially if it is their parent who accompanies them. Enabling young people who use specialised communication systems to interact with their peers, and form social relationships, can be especially challenging, because they depend on people being prepared to take the time to learn to use their method of communication. There are very few people who can use Fateha's communication aid, and thus very few people to whom she can talk directly. She can seldom join in with group discussions because the conversation moves faster than her communication aid. Her mother comments:

'Fateha was always the one with her hand up, wanting to have her say and share her ideas. Now, she can't do that. People say something, and by the time she's made her comment and got them to use her communication aid, the moment has gone, everyone else has moved on. Plus, she can't get their attention, they have to think of her having an idea to share, and children don't do that too much. Her carer has to say "Fateha wants to say something" and even if everyone stops and waits, it's just not the same. She has started to do a lot of writing because that's the way she can express her opinions and ideas, and figure out what she thinks, and make her plans, in a way that she can't with other people.'

It can also be very challenging practically for young adults who need long-term respiratory support to gain independence, because they often have less opportunity to leave the family home than their peers do. Fateha's mother explains:

'Fateha isn't going to be able to get a flat share and leave home, like she would have. In that way she will always be dependent on others. I am really determined that this will not fall on Farid, and she will have carers who will care for her, like she would herself if she could. So she will not be dependent on the family. She is still a smart kid, so she could study, but I think that it is unlikely that she will go away to university. Really there is no reason why she couldn't go away to study, because she will have carers, and my aim is for her to be able to live independently with them if she wants to, but it would be hard to organise. If she really wants to, I'm sure it is possible, but it would be hard for her to have a student life. She could live in another town, and attend lectures and everything, but the whole student scene isn't something that it will be easy for her to join in. You can't imagine her out clubbing or whatever.'

A part of the process of adolescents developing independence is their parents enabling this to happen. This can be more difficult for parents whose child needs long-term respiratory support than it would usually be, because they will have had to have a greater level of input into their lives, over a longer period of time, than other children require. Tom's mother recounts how:

'With Adam and Tom, you have spent their childhood really fighting this disease, watching out for every sign, getting treatment started, making sure they get the right things, and it is very hard to take a step back, and let them make the decisions. One time, I remember, Adam had a bit of a cold, and I knew we should get him onto antibiotics ASAP, get him to the GP to get them, etc., but he wanted to be in college that day for an event, and he was like: "Oh Mum, stop fussing." It was hard to let him make that choice. I had to, because he was 16 and it was his life, but it was very, very, hard to let go, or to let go enough but not too much. With my daughter, if I think she has a cold and should take a day off, but she says "stop fussing" it's easier to do, because the consequences are not the same. So it is harder to stop fussing and let a teenager who has health problems make their own choices or mistakes.'

One of the skills involved in working with children who need long-term respiratory support, particularly as they reach adolescence, is to work with them in a way that helps them to achieve the maximum independence possible, and to encourage others to do so as well. This includes facilitating their independence, whilst also valuing their parents' past and continued input into their lives, and supporting them, as well as their child, during the transition to independence (Department for Education and Skills and Department of Health 2006).

Leisure activities

Young people who need long-term respiratory support may find it difficult to join in the leisure activities that their peers enjoy. This may sometimes be because the activities themselves are not physically possible for them, but may also be because the venues in which the activities take place are not accessible. Tom likes spending time with his friends, but the places where they meet cannot all accommodate him: some have steps that he and his chair cannot negotiate; the toilets are not always accessible; and using public transport with his friends is challenging, because the buses are not guaranteed to be accessible, the spaces for wheelchairs are often full of suitcases, and trains have limited areas that can accommodate a wheelchair. His mother says:

> 'You can understand it: 16- and 17-year-old boys don't think about that kind of thing. They aren't going to plan out whether somewhere has steps or not, and you can't expect them to, but it does mean that Tom is left out. People are always telling us about accessible places where Tom can go, and they sometimes are good, but he doesn't want to go to special places with ramps and wide doors, and arrive by taxi. He wants to hang out with his friends, and get on the bus or train with them. It would be nice if most places had ramps and wide doors and accessible toilets so that he could do that. With the Disability Discrimination Act they should, but a lot don't. They are all "working towards" it, but when you are the one in the wheelchair today, "working towards it" isn't always very helpful.'

If facilities do not provide for those who have disabilities, they stop young people from being with their peers, and this may make them feel that they are less important or valuable than other people, which is unlikely to assist in the development of a positive sense of self-esteem. Whilst you cannot change society's provision for young people, you can perhaps help to facilitate support in a way that encourages the continuation of peer contact, enables young people to access the facilities they want to access, and makes clear that you feel they have an equal right to participate and a contribution to make. You may also be able to help them and their families to campaign for particular facilities to be made accessible.

Peer relationships are very important in adolescence: they give young people the opportunity to socialise and to develop the skills required to conduct adult relationships. Having the opportunity to develop peer relationships is as important for young people with additional health needs as it is for other adolescents, but their opportunities to meet their peers may be limited to times when someone is available and willing to accompany them. Having an adult with them may also mean that young people feel less able to express and explore their thoughts and ideas than their peers do (OFSTED 2010). Tom's mother comments:

> 'I am always happy at weekends and evenings to ferry him to where he wants to be, and wait for him, and so is his dad. But, at 16, you don't want Mummy and Daddy with you, or hanging around outside in the car waiting for you. That's not very cool, and Tom does want to be cool.'

As well as making the young person feel uncomfortable, the presence of an adult may change the dynamics of the group that they are with. It can be helpful if a person who is unrelated to them, or fairly close to their age, can be with a young person when they socialise, as this may make it easier for them to join in, and make their carer's presence less noticeable. Tom's mother recalls:

> 'Adam had one carer, Simon, who was great. If Adam wanted to meet his mates in the pub, Simon would take him there, and then go round to the other side of the bar and sit on his own, or chat to other people, and if Adam needed him, one of his mates could come and get him, or Adam could wheel over. So Adam was by himself with his friends, but he had someone nearby if needed. I hope we can find a Simon for Tom when he gets a couple of years older.'

When a young person has a condition that is deteriorating, they may find that friends and peers withdraw from them, both because they can no longer participate as they once could, and because their peers are unsure of how to cope with their increasing needs and long-term prognosis (Noyes 2006). Tom's mother has noticed that:

> 'As he has got less able, some of his friends have just dropped out. Maybe you could say they weren't friends anyway, but especially since Adam died, one boy in particular, I think, just couldn't handle it, and it was easier to cool off than deal with it. I can kind of see that, but for Tom, he lost his brother, and his best friend, and he knows that he is getting worse himself.'

Education

Although young people who need long-term respiratory support have the same right to education as other young people, if they have significant physical needs, their choices for post-16 education may be limited (Beresford 2004, Millar and Aitken 2005, OFSTED 2010). This may be especially so for young people who use specialised communication systems, and who need assistance with personal care. If local colleges cannot cater for them, they may have to make long journeys to access education, which brings with it the need for practical arrangements, and funding, for their transport to be agreed and organised (Millar and Aitken 2005).

It may also mean that any peer relationships that they have established at school cannot be continued at college. Although there is often funding available to help young people with additional needs to access education (for example, the disabled student's allowance), not everyone is necessarily aware of this or familiar with the system for claiming it (OFSTED 2010). One aspect of supporting young people may therefore be to help them and their families to work through the processes needed to help them to achieve their aspirations. You may also be well placed to work with staff in education establishments to help them to understand and meet the young person's needs. Fateha's mother comments:

> 'Even if she goes to the local university, we will have to do a lot of work with them, making sure everything is OK for her, that the facilities are OK, transport is available at the times she needs it, that she can access all the lectures and seminars, that there's somewhere for her to have her feeds, and be changed and everything. Getting her grades to get in and doing her coursework once she's there will be the least of her worries.'

Employment

Gaining employment is almost certainly more of a challenge for young people who have additional health needs than it is for their peers (Thornton 2003, Department for Education and Skills and Department of Health 2006). This does not seem to be because they lack aspiration or motivation to gain employment, but rather that, despite having similar levels of hope and aspiration to their peers, they fare considerably less well in the employment market (Burchardt 2005). This can make it very hard for them to sustain their motivation and hope, and may affect not only their employment and financial status but also their self-esteem. Tom's mother explains:

> 'I don't expect that Tom will get a job. Who is going to hire him? They would be worried that he wouldn't be reliable, and they would probably think training him was a waste of time. At the moment he is at college, which is lucky because that will take him to 18, and then we can see what he wants to do and how he is. For Adam, a job just never became relevant. But Tom has never even been able to get a Saturday job like his mates; he is limited in what he could physically do, but there are also not that many people who would take him on. His friend works in a sports shop, but when Tom went along with his friend and asked if they had any other jobs they just laughed. I don't think they meant to be unkind; they assumed he was actually joking. Imagine how Tom felt though. When you

look at what his friend does, Tom could do some of that: till work, advice on products, etc. It means he doesn't have that chance to earn extra pocket money and so he relies on us. We don't mind, but for his own self-esteem, it would be nice for him to be able to do something, like his mates do, and have that bit of independence – especially when his little sister now has a weekend job.'

In your work with young people it may be worth considering how you can help them explore their work options, and to think about what support they would need to make their hopes or aspirations become real. You may also be able to work with them to anticipate the concerns that potential employers might have, so that they can confidently discuss their ability to fulfil the roles they apply for, and clarify with employers how the support they would need could be organised.

Risk-taking

Risk-taking happens when someone voluntarily does something that creates, or is seen to create, a risk of losing something, but which also has the potential for some benefit. During adolescence, people are more likely to engage in risk-taking behaviour than at other times. A number of reasons for this have been suggested, including the physical changes of puberty, which create a drive towards excitement and adventure, developing more quickly than the cognitive-control system, which regulates these impulses (Reyna and Farley 2006, Steinberg 2007). Deciding whether a risk is sensible or not is also very individual; it depends on the relative value placed on what may be gained or lost. What one individual would see as reasonable risk-taking might be seen by another as unnecessarily reckless behaviour. In adolescence, the counterpart of the possible loss associated with risk is often the gaining of peer acceptance, which adults may not value as highly as young people do. Tom's mother explains:

'We know that Tom smokes and drinks with his mates, and we wish he didn't, but it is something he can join in with. There have been so many things he has tried to be a part of and can't be, that it is hard to say "No you can't do that", when it is the one thing that he feels makes him accepted, and part of the group.'

Although risk-taking is often seen as something negative, taking risks is an essential part of learning and developing independence. We all learn through experiencing successes and failures, and adjusting our behaviour and expectations accordingly (Stipek et al. 1992). Taking risks can help young people to develop their identity, understand how relationships work and how they will be expected to function in the adult world, and to take responsibility for their actions. Whilst some types of risk-taking are dangerous, or undesirable, finding out where the balance of risk-taking lies is an important part of young people's learning (Feldstein and Miller 2006, Sharland 2006).

It can, nonetheless, be harder for parents whose children have additional physical needs to allow them to take risks than it is for other parents. They may have to be physically present when their child takes risks, or at least tacitly agree to their risk-taking in a way that other parents do not. Tom's father comments:

> 'We know what they get up to because Tom has no choice but to get past us when he comes in. With a wheelchair and escort you can't really sneak in and crash out in your room. His mates probably creep in at midnight, and sneak past their parents, but Tom can't. So we have to decide whether to say something or really turn a blind eye, because we can't help knowing exactly what he does in a way that other parents probably don't.'

As well as a heightened awareness of the risks that their children take, parents have had to provide protection for their child over many years, and their knowledge of their child's condition can make allowing them to take risks more difficult than it is for other parents. Amelie enjoys all kinds of sports, and participating and being popular because of her sporting prowess is very important to her. She loves trampolining, but her mother worries about her falling off the equipment, being knocked out and stopping breathing:

> 'Another child who comes off the trampoline and gets a minor concussion is fine, but Amelie would stop breathing. It's the same with all the sports she does: gymnastics, swimming. You can't not let her do it, especially because that seems to be one of her ways of compensating for having CCHS and missing out on some things. As she gets older I suspect she will want to do even more dangerous things, and I have to learn to stand back and say: "Well, these are the risks, but you have to weigh them up and decide; just make sure someone knows what to do." That can be the hard bit though, because as an adult I think letting people know is no big deal, compared to the possible consequences of saying nothing, but already she doesn't want to, because she doesn't want to be different.'

Although it may be very difficult for parents, McConkey and Smyth (2003) describe the importance of allowing and enabling young people who have additional health needs to make decisions about what risks they see as worth taking. They describe how if young people are not allowed to take any risks, they may become lonely and isolated, and will not have the chance to learn how to make choices for themselves. Amelie's mother explains:

> 'I have to keep telling myself: she will have to manage her condition all her life, so my job is to be aware of the risks she is taking, including the risk when she doesn't tell people about having CCHS, and to help her to understand what the consequences might be. It's the same for my other daughter, really, but with Amelie the stakes are higher. If her

sister decides to experiment with alcohol and ends up unconscious, she'll be in trouble. If Amelie does that, and no one knows what to do, she'll be dead.'

Young people who have additional health needs may be unable to take risks as spontaneously as another young person would, and may have to depend on others to facilitate their risk-taking. This means that, as well as losing spontaneity, their risk-taking may be subject to uninvited comment and discussion in a way that their peers' is not. Some risks that they would choose to take may be unavailable because the person who would have to assist them is not prepared to be involved. Tom states:

'Maria [his carer] is pretty cool, she knows what we do, and she says it's up to me, as long as she isn't involved, as long as when she collects me I'm not smoking or drinking, then that's my deal. But the other guys don't have someone else who could approve or disapprove, or who they know knows and might tell their parents.'

Having to negotiate risk-taking with another person also means that the young person's 'success' or 'failure' in risky activities is known by another person in a way that it might not be for other young people. This risk may apply not only to activities that are considered dangerous, but to the risk associated with everyday events and rejection or acceptance in social situations. Tom's mother says:

'We have to drive Tom to most of the things that he wants to go to, so that means that he usually needs to check in advance if we are available. If it's a crowd of them going out, and it's a group decision, then that's fine, but sometimes I have felt sorry for him because he has to check with us before he starts to set something up, and then if it doesn't happen, or his idea doesn't work out, we know. Usually it wouldn't be like that.'

Young people's risk-taking can present legal or ethical challenges for staff, for example if a young person requests assistance to obtain non-prescription drugs, or engage in under-age drinking. Although you should accept a young person's right to take risks, you should be mindful that you are not, ever, obliged to break the law yourself in order to assist those you support. This may mean having to have very clear discussions with those you support, so that you remain non-judgmental, but do not compromise your own safety, or legal status, because of their choices. Tom's carer is very clear on this: 'Tom knows that what he does when he is with his mates is his choice and I don't stand in judgment. But I cannot be with a teenager who is doing drugs or drinking under-age. When he is with me, nothing illegal happens.'

Sexual expression

The development of a sexual self is a part of all young people's transition to adulthood, and a part of the young person's identity (Godfrey 1999, Nye 1999, McCann 2000, Earle 2001). Providing support for young people should therefore include consideration of their sexuality.

It can be very difficult for young people who need long-term respiratory support to have the opportunities for sexual expression and exploration that their peers have (Earle 1999). Many of the problems that these young people face in relation to their sexual needs being met are associated with other people's perceptions of them, rather than because their physical disabilities prevent them from engaging in sexual activity (Potgieter and Gadija 2005). Society often seems to regard people with impairments as not having sexual needs, and disabled people are therefore sometimes perceived as 'abnormal' when they express an interest in sexual activity (Shakespeare 1999, Earle 2001). Tom's mother explains:

> 'I don't think people expect Tom to have girlfriends. One person once said to me "Well, at least you won't have girlfriend trouble with Tom." The expectation is, he will not have a girlfriend. But why shouldn't he, really? At his age, when a lot of the boyfriend/girlfriend stuff only lasts a few weeks anyway, why write him off, just because he's in a wheelchair and he may not be here when he's 25 or 30? But no one thinks of him having a girlfriend, even though they often ask his sister, who is younger, about boyfriends. It is a bit insensitive really. People ask him how he is, how college is, but nothing about girls, and then, right in front of him, tease his little sister about whether she has a boyfriend.'

The opportunities that young people have for sexual expression may also be affected by their continuing to live at home, and being dependent on their families or carers (Sakellariou and Algado 2006). Tom has a carer at night to oversee his BiPAP and he has commented that some of his friends 'take girls home with them' but that he would have to '…announce to the carer that she needed to leave us alone for a bit, and then … have her there all night wondering what we got up to.' In addition, their physical limitations may mean that young people require assistance to be involved in sexual activities. This may include help with a range of activities associated with sexual need: getting information and advice, assistance to attend social events where they might meet potential partners, and assistance to experience sexual activity (Earle 1999). However, it may be difficult for them to ask for such assistance, and those supporting them may be unwilling or feel embarrassed to offer to help them. This may be especially difficult when the person in question is under-age. However, when you are supporting a young person, it is useful to make the distinction between what you are reluctant to help them with because of society's attitudes to sexual activity generally, and to disabled people having a sexual identity, and what is a real legal or ethical concern because of the person's age.

A further obstacle to young people being able to explore their sexual identity may be that their values and beliefs differ from those of the person from whom they need to seek assistance.

Whereas their peers would engage in whatever activity they wished to engage in, without requiring the approval or co-operation of a third party, young people who need physical assistance with their day-to-day care may feel fear or disapproval or judgment from others concerning their sexual desires. This is likely to be even more problematic if their sexual preferences are not in line with what society holds to be conventional (Earle 1999). For example, gay, lesbian and bisexual young people with disabilities may face particular barriers to exploring their sexuality (Abbott and Howarth 2007). When you are working with young people, it therefore seems helpful if you can make it clear that you are willing to discuss their sexual needs, and that, even if you cannot be involved in assisting them, you will not judge, or disapprove of, their desires.

Disabled people are more likely to rely on others for aspects of their day-to-day care, which creates an environment in which the risk of them being abused is increased (Cambridge 1999, Bernard 1999). People who have communication difficulties may also find it difficult to tell others about any abuse that they experience, especially if there are few people who understand the way that they communicate (Sant Angelo 2000). Whilst children and young people have the right to be protected from sexual abuse and exploitation, concern about this risk should not be confused with denying young people's right to a sexual identity. An atmosphere in which any evidence of sexuality or discussion thereof is taboo may, in fact, mean that young people have no forum in which they can discuss sexual abuse, and can increase (rather than reduce) the risk of it occurring.

Transition to adult services

As well as promoting young people's day-to-day independence, and supporting them as they move to adulthood, you may be involved in their formal transition from children's to adult services, and well placed to assist in making this a smooth process with a positive outcome. Achieving a smooth transition, and appropriate ongoing service provision, is important not just for the young person's adolescent years, but for setting them up for their adult life (Chamberlain and Kent 2005). As Fateha's mother comments:

> 'I think all the time about what needs to be set up for when she is grown up, because she could live to a good age, and I want her to have the best for her whole life, not just now. As a parent you are always trying to think what will best set your child up for life, and that is no different with Fateha. It just needs a lot more thought.'

Transferring from children's to adult services is a significant step for some young people, as it shows that they deserve the independence and respect that adult status confers. However, for the move to be achieved well, and to help the young person concerned to achieve their potential, the focus needs to be on what is best for the individual concerned, and how their aspirations, priorities and values can be catered for (Department for Education and Skills and Department of Health 2006). It requires good communication and collaboration between services, and for the young person and their family to be the central and guiding part of the process. It is also useful if the young person concerned has a trusted adult who can challenge and support them as they develop their ideas and decide what they most need and want, act as their advocate, and assist them in developing the ability to state their own needs (Department for Education and Skills and Department of Health 2006).

The right timing for a child's transition to adult services depends, amongst other things, on their developmental readiness, health needs and health status (Beresford 2004). Working out the best time to make the transition should be a joint decision involving service providers, young people and their families. Tom's mother describes how:

> 'Tom certainly does not see himself as a child any more. On the one hand he has wanted to leave children's services for a while, because he doesn't want the playroom and Winnie the Pooh on the wall when he's in hospital. On the other hand, he knows the staff on the children's unit, and they know him. We know his paediatric consultants really well, and although we do know the other consultants, we don't have that relationship with them, or the adult community nurses, or anyone. He is going to need his scoliosis sorting soon, and we decided that we want to go through the formal transfer to adult services after that, because that is going to be a big thing, and we all, including Tom, want to be working with people we know and trust. Everything is set up and we know who we will be working with, once he transfers, but we want the actual date to be after his surgery.'

Transition to adult services should ideally be planned well before the young person is ready to leave children's services so that the necessary co-ordination and negotiation can be achieved smoothly. This includes: identifying adult services that are willing and able to meet the young person's needs, deciding how the processes of information transfer will happen, negotiating administrative support, and ensuring the involvement of primary care, education and social care. Communication is probably the most important issue in achieving a smooth transition from children's to adult services (Department for Education and Skills and Department of Health 2006). The number of people and services involved means that having one named person for young people, their families, and all the services involved to use as the central point of contact and co-ordination is highly desirable. Such a person is often referred to as the Key Worker or Lead Professional (Department for Education and Skills and Department of Health 2006). Tom's mother explains:

> 'There are so many things to think about, the community teams, the hospital-based teams, the people he will see as an outpatient, doctors, physios, OTs, the social work

side of things, and his college. One of the nurses on the Children's Home Care Team has acted as our "Key Worker" and everyone knows that everything has to be fed in via her. If we hadn't had someone doing that, it would just be chaos I think, because no one would know what the others were doing and it would go round in circles.'

There are likely to be aspects of a young person's planning for and transition to adult services in which you can be usefully involved. This may include helping the young person and their family to explore what they need, want, and would prefer, and to decide how they can best explain their needs. Because you work with the young person every day, and are probably familiar with all the support they receive, you may be well placed to work with them to make sure that everything that needs to be put in place has been included in the plans for transition, and that the Key Worker is aware of every aspect of the support that they will need.

Summary

Young people who need long-term respiratory support have the same need to develop a positive self-image and independence as their peers. However, this may be much harder for them to achieve. They may find it more difficult to enjoy leisure activities and to mix with their peers than other young people do, and their opportunities for both education and employment may be reduced. They may also find it more difficult to experience and learn through risk-taking, and to explore their sexual needs. A part of your work may involve assisting them to have access to the opportunities and experience that their peers do, and to develop as much independence as possible. You may also be well placed to be involved in facilitating a smooth transition to adult services, and making sure that ongoing service provision is focused on meeting the young person's needs, priorities and aspirations.

Chapter 11

Children, families and loss

Children who need long-term respiratory support and their families may experience a sense of loss related to the same range of life events as everyone else, but they are also likely to have some losses that relate specifically to their health needs. What creates a feeling of loss, and how much a particular loss matters, is different for every individual, but having some insight into the particular losses that children and their families may feel can be useful.

Loss and children who require long-term respiratory support

The children you work with may have always had additional health needs. For example, James and Amelie have needed respiratory support since they were born, and Patryc has had a tracheostomy for as long as he can remember. There is sometimes an assumption that children who have always had a disability or disease do not feel the loss of what they never had, but this is often not the case. Amelie is sad that she cannot go to sleepovers with her friends. James gets angry and frustrated when he knows what he wants to do with his train track but has to explain this and get his mother to help him set it up correctly. Patryc wishes he could splash about in the swimming pool like other children do.

Children who have experienced a sudden and unexpected change in their situation, health and abilities are likely to feel the loss of what they no longer have. Fateha misses dancing, talking to her friends, and being part of the 'in' crowd. This is probably what causes her the most sadness – not being popular and surrounded by friends who she can chat to. Others, like Tom, gradually lose a range of abilities and grieve for what they have lost, but also for what they know they are likely to lose in the future. Children's losses may be highlighted when their peers achieve certain milestones that they cannot, or when people who are younger than them develop skills that they will never attain, or have lost. For example, Tom has seen his younger sister growing up and becoming increasingly independent as his own dependence increases. Specific events or rites of passage may also create particular feelings of loss: Tom's sister has just started a weekend job, whilst he has never been able to get a Saturday job and feels that he will never be able to work.

Although a child's health needs may create feelings of loss for them, the way in which other people or society as a whole treats them may also make them feel this way (Green 2007). This may include their degree of privacy and the respect that they are afforded changing or being different to that which their peers enjoy, and people's expectations of them altering. Fateha's mother explains:

> 'I think they mean to be kind, but when she manages to do something which, for her age, is very easy, people say "Oh well DONE!" When she actually has achieved something, then of course it would be good if people said so, but to say to her "Oh WELL DONE" or "That's RIGHT" when she tells the time or something is a bit insulting really. They never ask about her real achievements, so she never gets congratulated for things she actually has done well, but she gets this big commendation for simple things.'

A lack of facilities that cater for a child's or young person's needs can also cause them to experience loss. Tom's mother recalls how:

> 'Suddenly, when he got his wheelchair, he couldn't go to the local cafe where they all hung out. He was really unhappy, because he couldn't go out with his friends. He was well enough to, and wanted to go, but he couldn't get into where they went with his chair. He never asked them to move where they met, but I think he did feel upset that he wasn't important enough, for the cafe to cater for him, but also for his friends to think of changing their meeting place so that he could go. A couple of years later they did start meeting elsewhere, but he'd joined a different crowd by then – one that would have him, he said. They are not a crowd I particularly like him hanging around with, but he feels accepted there.'

As well as grief related to their own health or physical abilities, children are likely to feel loss if someone they know, with a similar condition, dies or has a significant change in their condition. Their grief may include sadness at losing the person concerned, but also an element of anticipatory grief, and heightening of concerns about their own illness, its likely progress, and their own mortality (Judson 2004). Tom's mother comments:

> 'When Adam died, we were devastated, because although people assumed we had come to terms with it, you never do. Tom was very quiet for a very long time after that. He has changed. His brother dying, [and] … knowing that he has the same disease. Until Adam went, we could pretend it wouldn't happen. Now we know it will, and he knows, and we know, that … next time it will be him.'

The range of events or situations that may cause children and young people to feel loss, and the number of occasions on which they feel this, can mean that they experience 'chronic sorrow'. This happens when the child never has the chance to adapt to their loss or address their feelings of grief before the next loss occurs (Eakes *et al.* 1998, Scornaienchi 2003). Tom's mother explains: 'Ever since he was diagnosed, Tom has had one loss after another, slowly losing his health, his friends, his dreams, his privacy, his brother.'

Loss for families

The families of children who need long-term respiratory support may feel loss of their own related to the child, or loss on behalf of the child. Their losses may relate to the expectations they had for the child; parents may lose the child they had planned, and planned for, and many of the experiences that they had expected to have with them (Barr and Millar 2003). This can include the time after a baby's birth being very different from their expectations, and their loss may relate to activities that they had expected to carry out, such as feeding the baby, bathing them, or taking them home. It may also relate to changes in their expectations of the emotional aspects of early parenthood; for example, losing the relaxed and happy time enjoying their baby that they had imagined. Aisha's mother recalls: 'The first few months were a nightmare. I had expected that with baby number three it would be busy, really busy, but fun. I knew what to do and expect, but she is so different, and we had no idea what was wrong and everything was a struggle.'

Families may also feel the loss of the usual responses and social markers that accompany a baby's birth; celebrations, cards and admiration may be replaced by awkwardness or sympathy. As their child gets older, their plans to socialise with their baby (for example, at parent and baby groups) may also be changed. Amelie's mother remembers: 'We missed all the mum and baby stuff because she was in hospital for so long, and by the time we came home I didn't feel like joining in, because my experiences were so different from everyone else's. I felt I wasn't a part of the "normal parents" any more.'

When a child's health status changes later in their life, their parents may experience feelings of loss or grief related to the child they had come to know, the plans they had for them, and the things they enjoyed doing with them. They may also lose their expectations, plans or ambitions for their child's future, education and employment. Patryc's mother explains:

'Patryc can do most things, but there are little things that I expected to do as a parent that I can't. Taking him swimming is more difficult. You have to be careful, he has to keep his trache above water, he can't splash around and he can't have swimming lessons because going underwater is part of that. Having a bath: he can't just splash around, you need to keep his trache in mind. He didn't learn to talk like other children do. It's small things that you expect without realising it.'

James's mother comments:

'I had this vague vision of being at the park with one crawling round on the grass and one in the swing; of them running out to the car and arguing over who gets in which seat. It's the small stuff that gives you a sudden shot of sadness, not the big things.'

Parents may experience ongoing and renewed feelings of loss as their child grows up, and they notice things that they cannot do, or ways in which their lives are different from other children's (Riesz 2004). Fateha's mother comments:

'When I see girls of about Fateha's age hanging around the school gates, chatting and messing around, I feel sad to think she will never be a part of that. She won't do that hanging round with her friends thing, which she would love. It's not just the big opportunities, the getting a job and going to university and getting married and having kids, it's the day-to-day things that make you feel sad.'

Parents may also feel a sense of loss over changes in their role because of their child's needs. Tom's mother describes how: 'Sometimes, you feel like all you do is give a medical handover; how his chest is, and all that. You never get to say "You know what, Tom is so funny. He makes me laugh," or complain about the state of his room. You never have a parent conversation. It's how well he is, what he can and can't do physically, and what he needs.'

Changes in parents' careers, financial security, home, lifestyle and leisure activities may cause them and their families to feel loss, as may alterations in their privacy and the way in which the family functions. They may also experience feelings of grief related to how society responds to their child. Fateha's mother comments:

'When we go out with Fateha, I hear people say "Oh what a shame" or "Poor thing" or whatever. With Farid they want to know what he's doing, but no one asks about Fateha. She is in the top group in her class in most things, but no one knows that because they don't see her that way. They don't even ask how she's getting on at school. Her achievements aren't celebrated, or even asked about.'

Children and young people who have a sibling with a genetic disorder may wonder about the impact of this on their long-term plans and relationships. It is useful for them to be able to discuss such concerns with someone who has knowledge of the disease in question, and it may be a part of your role to suggest this. Aisha's mother comments: 'SMA is genetic. So, although only Aisha is affected, the others might have the gene. When they think about having children, that will matter.'

Like the children themselves, families may experience chronic sorrow related to different aspects of loss in their lives and those of their children (Eakes *et al.* 1998, Scornaienchi 2003). Aisha's mother explains:

> 'Just as you think "OK, well I have got my head round that one, I can see that ... it'll be OK", something else comes along. It isn't always Aisha herself. I was just about getting my head around her dad leaving, then her diagnosis, what that meant for now and the future, that I had to leave work, the gastrostomy, CPAP, but then my other daughter's best friend moved away, and that really upset us both. It was perhaps a smaller thing, but it was the final straw, because it was a final bit of stability for Sarah that was gone, and I had relied on her mum a lot for helping Sarah get to things that I couldn't take her to. So it was the smallest of the things we had had to deal with, but it finished us off for a while.'

Like the children concerned, families may experience anticipatory loss, as they are often aware of the frailty of the child's condition, and the things they and their families will lose in the future. Green (2002) also describes how parents' loss is often complicated by the fact that the child who is associated with their loss is still a very real and important part of their lives. They are loved and valued for who they are, but their families' expectations for the children's lives and aspects of their own lives are lost. Whilst their grief does not diminish the parents' love for their child, the loss is still felt.

It may sometimes be assumed that when a child with long-term health needs, who has required considerable care, dies, their family will sense some relief. However, other family members are likely to feel the loss very strongly, on top of an already significant load of loss. Green (2007) points out that the exhaustion and challenges created by the practical tasks and barriers that parents face should not be confused with their feelings for the child as a person. For parents, losing a child with additional health needs still means losing their child. As well as loss of the child, families, and in particular parents, may lose a significant and often overwhelming part of their own identity, especially if they have spent a great deal of time caring for their child.

Some events may cause individuals or families to feel a mixture of grief and relief. If a child has had a long and difficult diagnostic pathway, their eventual diagnosis may be something of a relief, despite the loss associated with its finality (Nuutila and Salantera 2005). A diagnosis may represent the loss of hope that things would improve, or that nothing was actually wrong, but may also be a relief, in so far as a named problem has been identified, possibly clarifying the way in which it should be treated or managed. Getting a diagnosis may also sometimes mean that parents are provided with more appropriate assistance or support (Hewitt-Taylor 2007). Aisha's mother recalls how:

'When I found out that she had SMA, I was devastated, because of what it is, what it means, for her and for us, but in another way it was a relief to know what was wrong, what I was dealing with. It wasn't a diagnosis I wanted, because there is no treatment, no long term for Type I, but if that's what she has, then we need to know it, so that we can start to deal with it. '

Coping strategies

Grief is a solitary experience; everyone feels it separately and differently, even when those around them are also grieving. How individuals feel, and how they react to their feelings varies, and can affect them differently from day to day. Their feelings may be different, or more intense, at certain times, such as celebration times, life transition times, or at times that seem not to be any different from another but that have special resonance for them. Although there are no rules about how a person should grieve, or react to loss, thinking about how people may react can help you to understand the feelings of the children and families you work with.

People may not appear to feel loss, or to grieve, immediately after an event that we would think constituted a loss. This may be because they cannot initially understand or take in what has happened, and are perhaps finding it hard to organise their thoughts. They may instead react later on, as they begin to absorb the information. Other people may not appear to respond to loss because they only express their feelings in private, or with people they are very close to, or only when they are alone. Sometimes the combination of feelings that an event creates means that people's responses are very mixed. Aisha's mother recounts how:

'When we got the test results, and it was SMA, I think I sat there nodding my head and smiling … because I felt relieved that I knew what it was. I had an answer. It wasn't till I was in the car driving home that it suddenly hit me. This means she is going to die. I had to pull over because I started shaking. Aisha was in the back, and I dragged her out of her seat and just sat holding her. But when I got the news, I would swear I smiled.'

Loss may cause people to feel physical symptoms or sensations, including tightness in the chest or throat, breathlessness, lack of energy, over-sensitivity to light or sound, disturbed sleep and changes in appetite. It can be useful for people to know that it is not unusual to feel this way when they are experiencing loss, and it is not necessarily a signal of other physical or emotional problems.

People who experience loss are likely to feel sad, and to have an intense longing for what has been lost. They may feel sad about what they have lost, but this may also intensify the sadness they feel about other life events. Anger is also a common response to loss, but it may be felt about a variety of situations, not just things that are directly related to the person's loss. For example, if they have lost their expected experience of parenthood, or privacy, they may feel angry about you having to be with them to assist them, and things that would normally make a person slightly angry may make them very angry. Tom's mother describes how: 'Katie is cross all the time it seems. Part of that is probably just that she's a teenager but she gets so angry at the slightest thing. She gets really fed up about the carers being here, even though it hardly affects her, and if anything is just slightly wrong she reacts out of all proportion.'

Members of the same family may all respond differently to loss, loss may mean different things to them, and they may have different ways of addressing their loss. They may also experience the same feelings or have the same ways of managing their feelings as one another, but at different times and at different paces (Parkes and Markus 1998). This can cause conflict if individuals think that other family members are responding inappropriately or inadequately, do not understand their feelings, or do not care about the loss that the family has sustained. If a member of the family was involved in an incident that caused loss, their feelings of guilt about this, how other family members feel about and respond to the incident, and the support available to them will influence the way in which they manage their loss. This may also apply to genetic problems where one or both parents are affected, if this makes them feel responsible, or blamed, for their child's condition. Tom's mother explains:

> 'Sometimes I feel that people look at us and say: "After you had Adam, why did you go on and have two more?" But in fact we didn't know till after Katie was born that Adam had Muscular Dystrophy. We began to think something might be wrong at about three and a half, but he wasn't diagnosed till he was five – six months after Katie was born. I sometimes feel I have to explain that, because it seems as if we knew, and deliberately put Tom and Katie through this.'

The way in which grief and loss are experienced by individuals and within families may impact upon the family's functioning, and may lessen or worsen the stress that the family as a whole experiences because of the child's needs. Being aware of the different ways in which loss can affect people, and the many ways in which people respond to loss, may be helpful in assisting individuals to understand their own responses to loss, and those of other family members.

Theories of grief and loss

Although everyone is likely to suffer loss at some time, it is a very individual experience (Krueger 2006). It may nonetheless be useful to consider theories of grief and loss to guide you in the kind of support to offer. Whilst theories of loss tend to focus on experiences associated with death, they can also apply to the losses associated with a child having long-term health needs.

One theory of grieving is that of Kübler Ross (1969), who describes stages that an individual may experience following loss: denial, anger, bargaining, depression and acceptance. This model has been a useful guide for many people, and has helped them to gain some insight into what they and others feel following loss. However, the theory has been criticised for over-simplifying responses to loss, and suggesting a logical and linear progression to acceptance of what has been lost. Kübler Ross (1997) has herself clarified this by explaining that the stages are not intended to be seen as concrete, linear, sequential or easily definable. Rather, they are intended to give insight into what people may feel when they experience loss, and enable them and others to understand these feelings. Not everyone who suffers loss will experience all these 'stages', feel them in the sequence described, or move in a linear fashion between stages. Children with long-term health needs and their families are also likely to experience a range of losses and can thus potentially be at a mixture of stages for different losses. They may be angry about one loss, and remain so for some time, but find that they can more easily accept another loss, even if it occurs later on. This makes it difficult to define where a person is on a continuum of loss, and not necessarily particularly helpful. However, the concept of these different stages can be useful to help you understand the complexity of what people may be feeling.

Other writers see grief as requiring individuals to accomplish a series of tasks. Worden (1991) describes the tasks of accepting the reality of the loss, experiencing the pain of grief, adjusting to an environment without the person who has died (or, in the case of a child who needs long-term respiratory support, without the aspects of life that were known or expected), relocating the person who has died or the aspects of life that have been lost emotionally, and moving on with life. This type of model describes tasks, rather than stages, but still suggests a linear process, with a view to resolution and moving on, or from, what has been lost. However, it can be very useful in demonstrating that it is both realistic and necessary to expect people to feel loss very deeply, and to have to work on managing the feelings it creates, rather than moving smoothly through a process of adjustment.

Alternatively, rather than regarding adjustment as a linear process, individuals can be seen as having to create or find a meaning in their loss and rewrite what they had thought would be their personal story (Krueger 2006). This may mean searching for a reason for a child's condition, or a diagnosis to try to make sense of the situation, whilst also trying to understand what this means for them in the present and future. This may include not just what the individual or family expected to do or achieve, but the value that they placed on certain aspects of life, and what they thought they knew of other people, or society.

When a child develops a long-term condition, almost every aspect of their parents' life will require reconstruction (Rosenblatt 2000). As well as the initial impact of diagnosis, it is likely that, throughout their lives, they will come across situations or experiences that will not be as they had expected. The task of 'rewriting their expected life story' may therefore be a continuous one for children who need long-term respiratory support and their families. Fateha's mother describes a process a little like this:

'I was a PA in a large software firm, and the wife of a business manager, with two children who were doing well at school. Our house was the centre of all the action, for us and the children. We had friends round at least once a week, and there were always loads of children in the house. My life has changed so much you wouldn't recognise it. I am on my own now, and, although I do work, I work part time because Farid and Fateha both need me more, or I feel I want to be more available. In that way I have changed as a parent because, as well as my lifestyle changing, my attitudes and priorities have changed, I have decided to spend more time with the children and let work take a lesser place. We have enough money still, but we are more careful. I am not the mother of two popular high achievers. I'm the mother of a daughter who is very intelligent but has few friends or social options, and a son who prefers to go to his friends' houses rather than bringing them here. No one drops by here these days. I hardly ever socialise myself. So I am living a different life than I was. Just about every plan and part of my life is different. I won't be growing old with my husband, and I don't expect I will be attending my daughter's wedding or seeing her children grow up.'

Many theories focus on accepting loss, but if a person dies, Walter (1996) suggests that, rather than accepting the loss and moving on, those who are left behind need to integrate their memories of the person concerned into their continuing lives. Krueger (2006) suggests that individuals have to learn to love a person who has died in a different way from the person who was alive, but also be able to acknowledge the importance of that ongoing relationship. Providing opportunities for people who have been bereaved to talk about the person who has died can be a very useful part of supporting them, helping them to establish their ongoing relationship with them, and to rewrite their own and their family's life story (Davies 2004). It is often difficult for families to find people who are willing to talk with them in this way and it may be an important part of your role to enable them to do so. Tom's mother explains:

'Probably they just feel uncomfortable, and don't know what to say, but no one ever talks to us about Adam. If I mention him, there's an awkward pause and then the subject moves on. You know, no one ever even says "Yeah, he was such a great guy" or something, just to acknowledge that he was here. People often seem to want to get me to talk about how I feel about losing Adam, and about Tom's illness, but no one will talk about Adam himself.

It's as if he's been airbrushed off the family photos. The other day my nephew, who is only six, was round, and he said to me: "Auntie Mary, Adam did really funny voices. I wish he was still here to make me laugh." That was so sweet, it nearly made me cry. I said: "We all wish he was here, Toby." He said: "Yes, he was funny and his chair was cool." Just talking about Adam, as a person, not a loss, remembering him, was so good, but it took a six-year-old to do it.'

No one theory of loss is likely to be exactly right for all people, or situations. Loss and what it means for individuals, or families, is very complex and variable, and it is important that we work with people to achieve what will be helpful for them, not what any particular theory states.

Children's and young people's concepts of loss and death

Children feel the pain of loss as intensely as adults do, and also have to manage their feelings of loss (Riley 2003). A child or young person's level of understanding may not always be clear, but the assumption should be that everyone, regardless of their age or cognitive ability, can feel loss. Feelings of loss may in fact be worse for those who are unable to understand explanations or express themselves easily, because they may be less able to make sense of what has happened, or to ask questions and explain their feelings.

A child's feelings of loss or grief, and their understanding of death, will vary according to their age, cognitive level and previous experiences (Dyregrov 2002). Living with a long-term condition is likely to change a child's perceptions and insights, and often makes them more aware of issues related to loss than they would otherwise be at a given age. As with every other aspect of supporting children and families, one of the key aspects of working with children who have experienced loss is to focus on communicating with them and those who are close to them, and to be aware of how they may show their feelings.

When someone becomes unwell or dies, as well as missing them, or aspects of their life that their condition changes, children may feel guilty. They may feel that they have caused the event, or that their own or another person's illness is a punishment because of their behaviour or thoughts (Gilroy and Johnson 2004). Aisha's mother recalls:

'Sarah wasn't initially all that keen on the idea of another sibling. Then, when I had to explain about Aisha's illness to them, she said: "Is it my fault, Mummy?" I didn't know what she meant at first, but then I realised: she thought that by not wanting the baby she had somehow harmed her.'

Children may also think that by changing the behaviour that they feel caused the problem, or by some other action, they can reverse death or illness. Aisha's mother describes how: 'When I realised what she thought, I explained to her that Aisha's illness was nothing to do with anything she had thought, but she still kept asking me things like: "I was very good at school today, so do you think maybe Aisha will get better?"'

It can be useful to have some insight into what children may understand of death at different ages. This again differs from child to child, and is dependent on their experiences, but there are some rough guidelines below:

- Children under the age of five are not thought to understand that death is final, but they understand when someone is no longer there, notice when those around them are sad, and respond very strongly to this (Dyregrov 2002).

- Between the ages of five and ten, children gradually become aware of the finality of death, and that everyone will one day die. They begin to show compassion for other people's loss and to become concerned with injustice (Dyregrov 2002). This may include feelings about the injustice of their own or a sibling's additional health needs, the opportunities that they lose, or how people treat them, as well as the perceived injustice of death. They may feel angry about these things, and may display their anger in a variety of ways, not necessarily directly related to the loss in question.

- Children above the age of ten have a greater awareness of the longer-term consequences of someone dying than simply the loss of the person's immediate presence. They begin to reflect even more on justice, injustice, and fate and may also feel angry about this (Dyregrov 2002). Their developing independence may, nonetheless, mean that they are reluctant to share their feelings with others, especially with their family.

Tom's mother explains:

'I do worry about Katie, because she was so close to Adam, closer than she is to Tom. She always seems so self-contained, she used to talk to Adam, but she is quite distant from us. She never wants to tell us how she feels, but I know that since Adam died she has been really unhappy, and angry.'

Children, especially young children, may not seem to understand or take in news of loss, or may appear to carry on with their lives as if it is unimportant. This may be because they do not understand the finality of the loss (Dyregrov 2002), but also because, like many adults, they do not know how to respond. Like adults, they may experience shock and disbelief when confronted with loss, they may not take everything in at once, or know how to ask the questions that they have, or to explain their feelings. They may feel unable to cope with the way in which those around them are responding; and carrying on with their own activities may provide them with a sense of security when other people are behaving differently or in a frightening way. Children need the chance to think about what they have been told, or what has happened, to ask questions about it, and to share their feelings with people they trust.

Children's capacity to sustain or demonstrate sad emotions increases with age and maturity. If a child no longer seems sad following a loss, adults may believe that they have recovered from this. However, even when a child does not appear to be sad any more, they often are, or may return to their feeling of sadness. Responses to loss may become apparent months or even years after the event that caused them, and children and young people, like adults, revisit grief at different stages of their development and at particular times in their lives (Dyregrov 2002).

Some children who have suffered loss feel anxiety, experience vivid memories (for example, of the person who has died), have difficulty sleeping, or develop a fear of going to sleep. They may become clingy or regress in their development. Children may be scared by their reactions to loss, including times when they forget about their loss or the person who has died, and may need reassurance that this is to be expected, and not something they need to worry or feel guilty about. They may also need permission to play with friends and do the things that they always did. Tom's mother says:

> 'I had to make sure Katie knew it was OK to go out. I actually texted her best friend two weeks after Adam died and said: "It's OK to invite Katie out. We are getting back on our feet." Because people feel awkward.'

When children also have, or may have, the genetic disorder that a relative or sibling died from, they may have the very realistic fear that they too have, or will develop, this disorder and will also die. In some instances, they may know this to be the case. For example, Tom's mother recalls:

> 'When Adam died, what could we say to Tom? He has exactly the same disease, and he has been slowly getting worse, as Adam did. What can you say? We were all grieving for Adam, but we were also all avoiding the subject of what that meant for Tom.'

Supporting families who are experiencing loss

Whilst providing support in relation to loss is a part of your role, it is also important to recognise that families may have their own social support networks, which they might prefer to use. Some families may never want support from outsiders, and the time at which those who do want support value this most may not always be in the period immediately following a person's death or the discovery of a life-limiting illness. So, being aware of the losses that families may experience, and being available to support them, but also judging when and how this will be appreciated, is another key skill required in your work.

For all children, of whatever age, loss and grief are very individual experiences, but it is important for them to have supportive adults who are available to help them explore and make sense of their feelings (Gilroy and Johnson 2004). They may prefer to talk to an adult other than their parents about their feelings, and their parents may need to understand this, and to be helped not to feel rejected by their child, especially when they are also likely to be experiencing feelings of loss. Tom's mother comments:

> 'We realised that Tom and Katie probably needed someone they could talk to other than us. The term "counselor" was a real turn-off for them both. By luck, a friend had a guy lodging with them who was a bit older than Tom, but worked as a counsellor at a college for disabled children. He agreed to kind of "befriend" Tom, and just called by, offered to take him out, got his confidence and gave him someone to talk to. Because he wasn't afraid to bring up difficult subjects, I think he was good for Tom. We never knew what they discussed, but Tom enjoyed seeing him. He left the area a few weeks ago though. Katie, we are still trying to do the right thing for. Probably her friends and school are supporting her, and we try to, but she doesn't really respond to us.'

An important part of supporting children and their families is being aware that the things they may wish to discuss, the emotions they express, or their way of speaking may be difficult for you to manage. You may feel unsure about what to say or do, and what advice to give. Often, the only thing you need to do is be available, listen, and accept their feelings or thoughts. There will also be situations in which people need more assistance than you can offer, and your role may include highlighting this and suggesting other channels of support or input that may be beneficial to them. It can be useful to provide families with information on support groups, or organisations that offer support, which they can then access, or not, as they wish. These do not suit everyone, and may not meet a person's needs all the time, but they are an option that children, young people and their families may value.

When a child dies following a long-term condition, their family may need assistance and support regarding the practicalities associated with their death, some of which may be financial practicalities. Although a child's health needs often create financial difficulties for families, the child's death may sometimes worsen these problems. If their parents have been their main carers, they are likely to lose the financial allowances and state benefits that they received to help them care for their child. At the same time, they often have to meet funeral expenses and other costs, whilst already struggling financially (Corden et al. 2002). People who have been unable to work because of caring for a child with long-term health needs may find re-engaging with employment a slow and difficult process. Resuming employment will often be difficult because of their time out of the workplace, but also because they will be grieving at the same time as seeking work (Corden *et al.* 2002).

Where families have used support groups, they may feel unable to continue to participate after their child dies, and this, and other sources of support, such as schools or care staff, may be lost at a time when they would benefit from their input. It may be useful, in such situations, to help families identify new sources of support, such as alternative groups or services. When a child is expected to die, these possibilities can be sensitively explored in advance, so that families are able to prepare themselves to use new means of support if this seems likely to be necessary.

Summary

Children who require long-term respiratory support, and their families, may experience feelings of loss related to several aspects of their lives. They may experience repeated losses, and have little time to recover from each new loss. They may also anticipate the loss of things that they know will alter as the child's condition progresses. The responses of individuals and families to loss, and the ways in which they may wish to be supported, will vary, but being aware of the range of possible responses, and the reasons for them, can help you to support children and families more effectively.

Working closely with a family over a long period of time is a very different experience from many other types of care work. It can mean that you become much closer to children and their families and share a great deal more of their lives and experiences than you would in other situations, including feelings of loss (Samwell 2005). In the same way that families need access to support, it is important for you to know how and from whom you can seek support (Serwint 2004, Bartlow 2006). Although you need to achieve a balance between concern and over-involvement with families, you also need to acknowledge your own humanity and needs when you experience loss related to your work.

Chapter 12

Ethics and children's rights

When you care for a child who needs long-term respiratory support, there are almost certain to be times when you think about moral and ethical issues related to their care, or service provision. Morals are concerned with what is thought to be the right or wrong way to behave. However, because individuals, groups and cultures see different ways of behaving as 'right' or 'wrong', what is considered to be morally right can vary a great deal (Fletcher and Buka 1999). An ethic is sometimes defined as 'a set of moral principles' (Soanes *et al.* 2001), so ethics and morals are inextricably linked; and what is morally right and what is ethically right may often both be open to interpretation. Healthcare professionals all theoretically subscribe to the same moral and ethical principles, as laid down in their codes of practice, but how these principles are viewed and enacted by individuals may differ, depending on how each professional interprets them.

Ethical and legal aspects of practice are often discussed together, but they are actually two different things: the moral or ethical stance taken by an individual or profession may be different from the legal standards or laws of a country (McLelland 2006). Obeying the law of the country you are in does not guarantee that you are behaving in accordance with what you believe to be ethically right. Neither does following what you think is an ethically sound pathway guarantee that you do not break the law. For example, some people believe euthanasia to be the ethically right course of action in some instances. However, in the UK, this is currently illegal.

In healthcare, actions that promote health are generally considered to be moral and right, and those that produce the opposite effect are considered immoral (Wilmot 2003). It follows that healthcare staff are ethically bound to promote health. However, not everyone agrees on what constitutes health, or what the most important aspect of health is, so individuals' views on the ethically right course of action still vary. For example, some people might see it as ethically right for Aisha to receive CPAP at night, because this makes it easier for her to sleep comfortably, and appears to reduce the number of chest infections that she gets. Others might argue that, because she has a very poor long-term prognosis, the difficulty she experienced in adjusting to wearing a CPAP mask, and the distress this caused, was an imposition on her comfort and well-being, which could be considered unethical.

Sullivan (2003) suggests that the biomedical model of health, which historically dominated Western society, meant that health was viewed as a biological fact, with absence of physical disease seen as the ideal state of health. Interventions focused on the cure or reduction of physical ill-health have therefore traditionally been considered the morally or ethically right priority in healthcare. However, a broader view of health, which includes social, psychological, spiritual, cultural and emotional factors, is now generally accepted (Royal College of Nursing 2003). This means that we need a wider range of perspectives on what is beneficial, and makes it more complicated for us to decide on the ethically right course of action in relation to promoting health. It means that finding out what individuals see as 'health', and what they value in their health, have to play an important part in decision-making. Because it is unlikely that all individuals will agree on what constitutes 'health', making the 'right' decision can be very challenging. A child who requires long-term assisted ventilation may see good health very differently from a child who does not require assisted ventilation. How a child defines health may be different from how their family sees it, and what one individual sees as a priority in their health may differ from what others would see as a priority.

Because of the variety of ways in which people define health, it is very hard to prescribe what is and is not an ethical action. However, to help us make ethically sound decisions, or to consider all the ethical aspects of situations, it can be useful to use ethical principles or frameworks.

Ethical principles

Beauchamp and Childress (2001) describe the four main principles of medical ethics as being: beneficence, non-maleficence, autonomy and justice. These form the most common framework for debating ethics in healthcare.

Beneficence

Beneficence means 'providing benefit' so, in order to act ethically, you should act in a way that is beneficial to children and their families (Wilmot 2003). However, because not everyone agrees on what is beneficial for children and families, the definition of an ethically sound action remains open to interpretation. It also means weighing up what aspects of benefit matter the most. An intervention that has some benefits may also have some negative outcomes or risks. For example, James's mother has decided that she will try to let him enjoy activities that he likes, rather than constantly worrying about whether she is doing exactly the right thing with his treatments. She says:

'I have been known to decide to miss out doses of his inhalers, or not be so diligent with his oxygen delivery, if it means he is going to have fun. You have to constantly weigh up, with a child like James, what matters the most. Is it being as well as he can be physically, but cocooned at home, making sure he has oxygen every minute of the day, avoiding every infection; or out and about taking his chances, but living, laughing, enjoying what he has?'

Many actions or decisions are not wholly beneficial or harmful, but a balance of benefit and harm should be sought in which the likely outcome is weighed in favour of benefit rather than harm.

Non-maleficence

Non-maleficence means 'avoiding causing harm', so you should act in a way that does no harm to those you support. Although this sounds logical and straightforward, determining what is harmful is not always any easier than determining what is beneficial. It includes thinking about physical, social, emotional, spiritual and psychological harm and also sometimes means balancing whether harm caused in one respect is outweighed by harm averted in another. For example, Aisha's mother recalls how, when she first began to have CPAP, she found the mask very uncomfortable and difficult to sleep with:

'She hated it, and for the first two weeks I really did wonder if I was doing the right thing. She got a very sore face, and cried every time I put it on, and couldn't get to sleep … but we kept going. At times I thought "Why am I doing this?" but now she is fine with it. We got a different mask that fits OK, we have got used to putting it on, and she is much better with it than she was without it. She is happier and more settled and getting fewer infections, so now I think I made the right choice, but it was a difficult one, because it did cause her distress, and discomfort.'

As well as the complexity of deciding what is beneficial or harmful to a child, the effect that something which is beneficial to them has on their siblings and parents has to be included in debates over what is ethically right (Menahem and Grimwade 2003). Aisha's mother comments:

'Sometimes, we all look at Aisha, and say that we need to do something because she needs it, but I have three children, and they all matter. Of necessity, I sometimes focus more on Aisha, but I value them all equally. The other week someone told me about one of those multi-sensory places where Aisha could go. Another mum is taking her daughter every week. That would be great for Aisha, but it is a one-and-a-half hour drive each way, and it would mean that I had to get someone else to collect the others from school, and that I got back late, and still had everything else to do, which would mean I had less time with them. I already squeeze in little enough time with them, so I have decided that I will only go when they are doing something else anyway. That will be very, very, occasionally, but everyone has to be put into the equation. It would be great for Aisha to go every week, but it would not be great for the other two, so we have to find a fair balance.'

Respect for autonomy

Autonomy is defined as a person's ability to make self-determining choices (Lowden 2002). The ethical requirement to promote autonomy therefore means that you should aim to enable those you support to make their own independent choices about every aspect of their lives.

Although respect for autonomy is now a popular ideal in society as a whole, as well as in healthcare, this has not always been the case (Joffe et al. 2003, Sullivan 2003). Traditionally, medical staff decided what treatment, care or interventions a patient should receive, and it was seen as unreasonable to impose any burden of decision-making about their health on individuals (Kennedy 2003). This was partly because of the prevailing belief that 'health' meant physical health, with medical staff therefore being considered to have the best understanding of what would achieve this. With the acceptance of a broader view of health, the importance of individuals being able to make their own decisions, based on what they see as health and what matters most to them, is now recognised (Lowden 2002, Kennedy 2003, Wilmot 2003).

In order to make autonomous decisions, people need enough clear, accurate and unbiased information about the matter in question, the opportunity to express their choices, and to have these acted upon. Providing sufficient information in a way that people can understand may be difficult in any situation, and can be even more challenging with children, where those involved have different cognitive levels from what would be expected at their age, or where they have communication difficulties. If a child uses a special communication system, their speech is difficult to understand, or their hearing or sight is impaired, the systems that they use to communicate must be available when discussions are taking place, which concern them. A person who can assist them, interpret their communication or act as their advocate may also need to be present during discussions, and it is important that a child's level of understanding and ability to make decisions is not confused with their ability to communicate verbally, or their physical health. Fateha's mother comments:

'Although Fateha is still quite young, she is bright and she wants to know what is happening, and understand why, and have her say. Our paediatrician is great: she always explains things to Fateha, and listens to what Fateha wants to ask, using her communication aid. But one neurologist we saw was dreadful. Fateha wanted to ask a question and, because it takes time for her to ask, this woman just said: "Well, Mum, find out what it is that's bothering her and maybe check with your GP, or ask me at the next appointment." I was furious, and so was Fateha. She wouldn't have said that to a child of Fateha's age and intelligence who wasn't disabled in the way Fateha is.'

Autonomy relates to every aspect of a person's life, and, as well as making sure that the children and families you work with have enough information to make choices about what seem to be major issues, they also need to be given information and opportunities to make as many choices as they can about every aspect of their lives. This may be about small everyday things, such as what they want to do or wear, or major things such as whether or not they want a new type of medical treatment, or surgery. Fateha's mother explains:

'At Fateha's school, they don't have uniform, so it's a bit of a fashion parade, and Fateha cares what clothes she wears. I think people sometimes forget that, but just because she is disabled, doesn't mean she wants to go to school in last year's clothes. I ask the carers to let her choose what she wants to wear each day, and to let her see if she likes how it looks on her, if she wants to.'

Although people need to receive unbiased information in order to act autonomously, it is hard not to let the information that you give be influenced by your interpretation of it. When you are discussing choices with children and families, you need to be very aware of your own beliefs, values and experiences, and how these may influence what you encourage others to do. This does not mean that you should pretend that you do not have views of your own, but rather that you should acknowledge what these are, so that the people you work with are clear about how they may influence the discussion. It is also useful to be able to direct people to alternative sources of information, so that they have the chance to hear a range of views and opinions.

Fateha's mother also describes how children's decision-making can be complicated by the fact that they need to be subject to the usual range of parental rules:

'I lay the ground rules with Farid and Fateha: what is and isn't OK to wear, or say, or do, but with Fateha, because her carers are with her and often have to do things for her, I have to make sure they know the ground rules too – like no jeans at school. I don't let either of them wear jeans to school, so although Fateha can choose what she wears, and I expect her to be given that choice, the carers need to know what she is allowed to choose within. Whether they think it's OK to wear jeans to school is up to them, but my rule is: no. Any other child has that "choices within the rules" thing, and Fateha is no different.'

Although autonomy involves independence, promoting autonomy does not mean leaving a person unsupported, to make their own decision. An autonomous person can accept support and assistance from others, and may decide to take the opinions of others on board and act on these, but this must be their choice, rather than it being imposed on them (Kaplan 2002, Lowden 2002). James's mother states:

> 'I expect to be in charge of the decisions about James, because he is my son. That doesn't mean I expect to have to know everything though. One time when he had begun to have more seizures we saw the neurologist and he said that he thought we should try a new drug. He explained what it was, and how it worked, and about the side effects, and I agreed. In that situation, I didn't feel I needed to go and look all the options up, because this is a man I trust, and it sounded sensible, so I decided to go with it. Sometimes I will argue the toss with the doctors, or ask them about other options or things I have read about, depending on what it is, who it is, and how I rate them, but usually I trust this particular doctor's judgment and go with what he suggests.'

Whilst promoting autonomy is an ethical obligation, those who make autonomous decisions are also responsible for these, and the outcomes of their decisions. This applies to health as much as any other area of life and is one reason why the decisions that people make have to be truly informed. James's mother explains:

> 'I need to be given accurate information because it is me who has to live with what I decide. I decided to stop James's tube feeds, and, although it creates problems, I chose that, because I thought it was the best option. I still stand by my choice, but that is why I need all the information, so I can choose and take responsibility, knowing what will probably happen because of my choices, for James, but also the whole family.'

Decision-making is also very difficult where there is little certainty. The speed at which medicine and technology advance means that options that will be available in years to come are often largely unknown. The complexity and rarity of the medical problems that some children have also means that it is almost impossible to be certain about the outcomes of certain treatments or interventions. Where there is uncertainty, there should always be truthful and clear discussion of the knowns and unknowns, and the relative risks of any treatment or intervention that is being considered, so that these can be weighed up in the decision-making process.

Promoting and respecting an individual's autonomy does not mean that support or caring should be withdrawn from the decision-making process (Orfali and Gordon 2004). Rather, it makes supportive and non-judgmental facilitation of decision-making necessary, with understanding and compassion after the event, as individuals and their families live with and review their decisions, often in the light of evidence that was not available to them at the time when the decisions were made.

Justice

Although it is important to consider whether or not you are doing good, doing no harm, and promoting the autonomy of the children you work with, the wider picture also has to be considered. Actions almost always have implications beyond the person to whom they are directed and the principles of preventing harm, doing good, and promoting autonomy have to be seen alongside the requirement for justice (Grace 2001). The team that provides Aisha's night care currently has two staff on long-term sick leave, and one vacancy, in a team of ten. They have had to cut back on all provision and use agency staff to cover as many shifts as possible. This means that Aisha, who used to receive night care and one weekend in four 24-hour care, now gets no day care options at weekends, only night care. The team manager explains:

> 'I know it is hard on her mum, because she has two other children and she is on her own, but we have had to try to be fair to everyone. Everyone is getting less, and we have had to decide what it is fair to reduce, across the board. If I just looked at Aisha and her family, and had unlimited funds, I'd probably offer her 24-hour care, seven days a week, but I haven't. If I give her more, someone else gets less. It is hard on families, I know, but I don't have an unlimited pot of money or staff.'

The problem of allocating resources fairly is very complex because what health means for individuals, what needs each individual would prioritise, and how they would want these to be met, vary. For example, Aisha's current care package is for night care, from 8 pm until 8 am, seven nights a week. However, her mother has suggested that, since the reduction in staffing, she would prefer to have day and night care one weekend in four, and give up one night of care provision a week, which she could cover. However, fitting her request in with the requests of other families, and staff availability, is problematic. The manager of the team in question says:

> 'I am trying to sort that one out, because it is reasonable. She isn't asking for extras – in fact it would be less hours in total – it's just a different pattern. But although it sounds easy, when everything is finely balanced, as it is just now, moving a bit of one care package has implications for the others. So although in one way we do want to give families choices, when it comes to the nitty gritty of achieving that, it isn't always so easy to do.'

Deciding on a fair way to share out resources is never easy, and, as it becomes possible to manage more and more complex health problems, the question of how to provide equal services for all, using a finite national budget, becomes very difficult (Boosfeld and O'Toole 2000, Poses 2003). National Health Service resources cannot meet everyone's needs as quickly as they would like, or to the ideal standard. It would therefore be desirable to have some agreed way of deciding what will and what will not be provided, and what standard is deemed to be reasonable. However, because there will never be agreement between all interested parties on what constitutes a reasonable standard, and which aspects of health should take priority, the task of deciding what is 'fair' is extremely challenging.

Utilitarian principles are often used, or described as being used, to decide on how finite healthcare resources should be divided fairly. This means taking an approach based on the principle of the most productive use of resources and the achievement of the greatest good for the greatest number (Draper and Sorell 2002). Using this utilitarian approach, justice would require that healthcare resources be used in a way that creates the greatest good for the greatest number of people or uses resources most productively overall. However, this does not simplify the debate on resource allocation, as it still requires us to define what is good and what is productive. Using purely utilitarian principles, some people might say that sustaining Aisha's life and quality of life by using CPAP was not justified, because her long-term prognosis is poor. However, her family would probably not agree, and would see the additional time that they gain with her, and her improved quality of life, as productive and good for them as a family, as well as for Aisha.

Another approach is to use deontological principles, to judge an action solely on the benefit of its own outcome, separate from any broader consequences. This approach places the individual and their well-being centrally, and, in Aisha's case, would probably favour the opposite viewpoint from the utilitarian approach. The benefit of her having CPAP is that her quality of life, and the time her family has with her, is improved, and this makes it ethically right from a deontological perspective to provide CPAP. However, this argument does not necessarily meet the requirement for justice, where the resources allocated to one person inevitably impact on the resources available for others.

Clearly, the four ethical principles of beneficence, non-maleficence, autonomy and justice do not always provide easy answers to ethical dilemmas, and a combination of utilitarian and deontological reasoning is often apparent in decision-making. However, these principles can provide a useful framework for debating ethical issues. They can help you to think about whether actions taken by yourself or others can be considered 'ethical', and enable you to appreciate the complexity of the decisions that have to be made.

Duties of veracity, privacy, confidentiality and fidelity

The four ethical principles of beneficence, non-maleficence, autonomy and justice are often discussed alongside the four generally agreed duties of healthcare professionals. These are: veracity, privacy, confidentiality and fidelity (Beauchamp and Childress 2001).

Veracity, or truth telling, is based on the principle that respect is owed to others and that a part of respecting people is telling them the truth (Beauchamp and Childress 2001). Veracity is also linked with the requirement to promote autonomy because, unless a person is told the truth, they will not be receiving accurate information on which to base their decisions about their own lives. If a person cannot rely on being told the truth by another person, they cannot trust them and thus the requirement for fidelity, or trust, is also affected.

The requirement to tell the truth means not only that what you say should be literally true, but also that you have a responsibility to ensure that it is said in a way that makes its meaning clear, and difficult to misinterpret (Kirklin 2007). James's mother recalls:

> 'Often when he was a baby, but even now, I ask about his future, or something, and get an answer that is basically fobbing me off. I remember one time, when he was in the neonatal unit, asking a doctor what he thought the future held for James, and he said: "Well, he's doing OK, we think he'll be OK now." I took that to mean he would be OK, like other children, not that he would still need oxygen at the age of three, and be tube-fed for years, and not be able to walk. OK to me means the same as Alice, but OK to him meant he wouldn't die, and would get home. I wouldn't say he was lying, but we weren't talking about the same thing when we said: "OK".'

As discussed in Chapter 2, everyone has a right to privacy (Council of Europe 1950, McLelland 2006). When you work in the home setting, you are likely to have access to a greater quantity of private information than you would in other settings, as mentioned in Chapters 2, 6, 7 and 8. The child's, young person's and family's personal privacy, and privacy about their health-related information, should all be respected. Closely linked to respecting a child's and family's privacy is the requirement to maintain confidentiality.

Maintaining confidentiality means that you should not unnecessarily disclose any information about the families you work with (McLelland 2006, Nursing and Midwifery Council 2008). Individuals have a right to make their own decisions in every area of their lives, and who should have access to information about them is no exception. They themselves are also in the best position to understand the implications of information being disclosed (McLelland 2006). Aisha's mother recounts:

> 'It is amazing how information spreads. One of Aisha's carers once mentioned to a friend of hers what I had bought Kyle for his birthday. By coincidence, this friend had a child at the same pre-school as Kyle was in, and somehow the boy got this information and my son came home knowing about his big treat. I was furious really. I know it's a small thing, and I'm sure she didn't realise what she was doing, but that is how you get to feeling that the whole world knows your business.'

There may nonetheless be exceptional circumstances, where the requirement to respect confidentiality can, and should, be overridden (Nursing and Midwifery Council 2008). These include statutory exceptions (such as the notification of certain infectious diseases), where child protection is an issue, and in the public interest (Dimond 2005, McLelland 2006). Nevertheless, if you are given information with the expectation that it will be confidential, and realise that it cannot be kept confidential, the person concerned usually needs to be made aware of this, unless doing so will jeopardise your personal safety or that of others. This includes situations where you feel that you must disclose information that children share with you to their parents (Dimond 2005).

The relationship between you and the child and the family you work with should be, as mentioned in Chapter 3, one of trust (McLelland 2006). This includes giving information that is trustworthy, and fulfilling the trust that the child and family have that their privacy and right to confidentiality will be maintained. Fidelity is also concerned with faithfully maintaining your duty of care, and fulfilling the trust that people place in you. A breach of any part of your duty of care, or of any ethical requirement, can be seen as a breach of your duty of fidelity.

Consent

One aspect of care that often creates ethical and legal dilemmas for healthcare practitioners is consent, particularly when working with children and young people. Consent to treatment or care is usually linked with the ethical obligation to respect autonomy, because valid consent requires an individual to have been given information about the decision in question, to have understood and considered it, and to have made the decision to agree to whatever they are consenting to. A great deal of information on consent relates to interventions such as surgery, or investigations carried out in hospital. However, gaining consent should be a standard part of the support that you offer children and families, and you should be sure that the person concerned consents to anything that you are doing for or with them (Nursing and Midwifery Council 2008). This type of consent is often quite informal, but whenever it is possible for the person concerned to express their wishes, you should check whether or not they agree to what is happening.

Working with children, and especially children who have additional health needs, often brings into question the issue of who can or should give consent. The major point in such situations is not the child's state of health, or their age alone, but whether or not they are competent to make the decision.

Competence relates to a person's ability to perform specific tasks. To be competent to make a decision, the person concerned must be able to make that particular decision. To achieve this, they need to have enough information about the decision in question, and to have this presented in a way that they can understand. This includes the reasons why whatever is being suggested is thought to be necessary, the likely outcomes, and any alternative options. They must also be given the opportunity to ask questions and discuss the options involved (Lowden 2002). If information is provided in such a way that a person cannot understand it, their ability to achieve competence will be reduced, but this is not the same as a person not being able to be competent. It means that whoever is giving the information, through their actions or omissions, has prevented the person from becoming competent, and this is unethical, as it means that the person's right to autonomy is not being respected. You are not, however, solely responsible for being able to explain everything to everyone. There are likely to be times when you do not have enough information, or cannot make yourself understood, and have to seek help and advice from other people, and work with them to provide explanations that a child or their family can understand.

If a child is competent, the principle is that they should be allowed to consent to health-related care and interventions. This principle applies equally to a child who requires long-term respiratory support. The fact that children may need things to be explained in a different way to adults, or by using a particular method of communication, does not mean that they are not competent to make decisions. It means that an effort has to be made to provide information in a way that they can understand (Watson et al. 2006).

Although children's autonomy and right to consent to treatment or interventions is recognised, their legal rights in this respect are not as clear as this might suggest. According to the Children Act (Department of Health 2004c), children should always be consulted (subject to their age and understanding) and kept informed about what will happen to them. However, when a child or young person can consent, or, perhaps more importantly, withhold consent, to treatment, care or interventions, is not completely clear.

In the UK, children under the age of 16 do not have a statutory right to give consent to treatment. However, the House of Lords has ruled that if a child understands the nature of a proposed treatment, and its effects, then they can be considered competent to consent (Gillick vs Norfolk and Wisbech Health Authority 1986). This has been termed 'Gillick competence', and the guidance that was given by Lord Fraser during this case is referred to as the 'Fraser Guidelines'. Whether a child is considered to be competent to consent therefore depends on when they are able to understand the decision in question and its likely consequences (Parekh 2006). This stage may be reached by different children at different ages, and a child may be competent to make some decisions, but not others, depending on their understanding of the matter in question.

The issue of a child's competence to consent can be complicated when they have long-term health needs because, regardless of their age and cognitive level, their experiences may mean that they have a better understanding of health-related matters than their peers, or even some adults who have had limited healthcare experience. If a child's competence to consent is in question, legal and medical personnel are often asked to assess this. However, Parekh (2006) suggests that a wider range of professional groups, and those who know the child best, should be involved in such an assessment. This may be especially important for children with long-term health needs; those who have worked closely with them, or who are familiar with their methods of communication, may be best placed to ascertain their views and to decide whether they have been able to access, understand and weigh up all the available information when making their decision. Your input may be critical in working with others to help the child or young person to achieve their maximum level of competence, and to assist in assessing this.

The Family Law Reform Act (1969) states that 16- and 17-year-olds have a statutory right to give consent to medical, surgical and dental treatment. However, parents can also give consent on behalf of a child up to the age of 18. This means that, although a 16- or 17-year-old can agree to treatment, if they refuse treatment this can be overruled by their parents or by the courts if it is felt to be in their best interests (Dimond 2005). Thus, although children who are deemed competent can consent to treatment, if they are younger than 18 and they refuse treatment, their parents may consent on their behalf, or the courts may overrule their refusal if this is deemed to be in their best interests (Parekh 2006). Until the age of 18, children and young people are therefore not fully autonomous in decision-making about their health, as they can consent to, but not necessarily decline, treatment (Lowden 2002, Parekh 2006).

The value of allowing a child to consent without allowing them to withhold consent is debatable, because it essentially means that consent is no more than the right to agree with others. In practice, children's views and opinions may well be taken into account, and their refusal to consent is likely to be respected. However, in law, there seems to be no obligation to accept their refusal to consent to treatment, particularly if this is not in accordance with their parents' wishes, or society's views on what is in their best interests.

The aim of consent processes should be to help people to make informed choices, not to coerce them into agreeing to any particular course of action. Nonetheless, if a child or young person withholds consent, it is important to find out what they are refusing, and why – for example, to check whether their reluctance is about the procedure being proposed, the outcome of the procedure, or both, and whether they are declining at this point in time, or refusing in principle. Fateha's mother describes how:

'One of the carers is very good about checking what Fateha wants, but even then you have to be a bit careful. One time she told me that Fateha didn't want a shower, so she wasn't having one. So I went along like the Big Bad Wolf and asked Fateha: "Do you actually want to go to school without a shower and without having your hair done, which is what will happen if you say you won't have a shower, or do you just mean you don't want to get out of your warm cosy bed?" I know it seems a bit mean, when she has so much to put up with, but actually she did want to go to school showered and looking pretty. She just didn't want to get out of bed, like most of us.'

Rights

As well as the ethical principles that you should work within, the support that you provide should uphold the rights of the children and families with whom you work. Rights are essentially rules of interaction between people and, as well as protecting people, they place constraints on the actions of individuals and groups. For example, if we all have the right to be heard, this also means that we are all obliged to listen to others.

In order to be of any value, rights have to be recognised. If you believe that the child you work with has a right to be able to access the local toy shop, for you to be able to insist upon this right being met, the toy shop owner also has to recognise, or be required to recognise, this right. In many cases, the rights of individuals and groups have been enshrined in law, in order to make expectations clear. What constitutes reasonable behaviour might seem obvious, but unless there is a clear standard by which we can define what is considered to be right, it is very hard to prove that a person or an organisation has acted unreasonably, or for organisations or individuals to know what they should do in order to be considered to be acting reasonably. Acts that state what are deemed to be reasonable expectations can therefore be very useful.

The Human Rights Act, as its name suggests, outlines the rights that all human beings are entitled to, and the way in which all people can expect to be treated. This came into force in the United Kingdom in 2000 (HMSO 1998) and it is therefore expected that the rights outlined in the act will be met in the UK.

Children's specific rights are also recognised (Office of the United Nations High Commissioner for Human Rights 1989, Department of Health 2004c). The United Nations Convention on the Rights of the Child is intended to give children worldwide an equal right to certain standards of life and safety (Rowse 2007). Although the convention itself is not legally binding, it has been ratified by the British government, which means that it can be used as an argument in British law (Rowse 2007). By ratifying it, the British government has agreed to do everything possible to implement it, and to monitor whether or not the convention's principles are observed (Dimond 2005). The Children Act (Department of Health 1989, 2004c) provides a legal basis for the enforcement of some parts of the convention.

The Disability Discrimination Act 1995 (HMSO 1995) and its successor the Disability Discrimination Act 2005 (HMSO 2005) are intended to counteract discrimination against people because of any disability that they may have. They define disabled people's rights in the areas of: employment, education, access to goods, transport, facilities, services, and buying or renting of land and property. The Disability Discrimination Act 2005 (HMSO 2005) states, amongst other things, that disabled people have the right to expect to be able to use public transport easily, to have access to everyday services and facilities, and that service providers must make reasonable adjustments to enable people with disabilities to access and use their facilities. The act also requires service providers to cater for a full range of disabilities and access needs. A hotel cannot limit its provision to meeting the needs of people with impaired sight and claim to have met the requirements of the Disability Discrimination Act; it also has to take into account people with, for example, speech, hearing and mobility problems.

The Disability Discrimination Act (2005) and the Special Educational Needs and Disability Act 2001 (HMSO 2001) make it unlawful for education providers to discriminate against disabled pupils or students, place duties on schools not to treat disabled pupils less favourably than others, and require them to make 'reasonable adjustments' to ensure that they are not disadvantaged. The Disability Discrimination Act applies to extracurricular as well as schooltime activities, and means that children who have disabilities should be enabled to participate, if they wish to do so, in all the activities associated with school life that are open to other children. However, sometimes it can still be difficult for children's rights to be met, unless all services work together to achieve this. Fateha's mother explains:

> 'Her school is very good. They *do* make things available to her. Often it is the other things, like transport, that don't kick in. They have made sure she can get everywhere in the school, and have worked really hard with us on including her. They were more than willing to make sure she could go to chess club after school, but we had a problem with transport and staff handover times with that one, so it didn't happen, but it wasn't the school's fault.'

The Equality Act (HMSO 2010) aims to clarify and simplify the law related to discrimination and inequality. It addresses various elements of equality, including people's right not be discriminated against on the basis of disability, and includes their experiences in schools, further education establishments, employment and everyday service provision. It also increases the protection that carers have from discrimination because of their caring role. It is therefore relevant to many children who require long-term respiratory support, and their families.

Safeguarding children

Children have a right to protection from harm, and their welfare is always paramount in all decisions concerning them (Office of the United Nations High Commissioner for Human Rights 1989, Department of Health 2004c). It is important for you to be aware of local procedures for safeguarding children, and to follow these in any case where you are concerned. However, although there are situations where something is very clearly harmful to a child, there are also times when individuals' views on what is an acceptable way to treat children may differ. This is one reason why you should be aware of the child protection processes, procedures and resources that are available, and the channels for discussing concerns and seeking advice on the best course of action as well as for reporting abuse.

It is especially important for you to be aware of safeguarding issues when you work with children who have some degree of disability, because disabled children are more likely to experience abuse than other children, and may be less able to report this (Department of Health 2004b). If a child has communication difficulties, they may find it difficult to report abusive behaviour, especially if there are not many people they can communicate with, or if they communicate mainly through the person who is mistreating them. Society's attitudes to disabled children may make it difficult for them to find someone who will listen to, or believe them, and behaviours that are associated with the abuse a child is suffering may be wrongly attributed to their disabilities.

Receiving care from a number of individuals can make it difficult for children to set and maintain boundaries with staff, and can create opportunities for abusers (Department for Education and Skills 2006). Some ways in which the risk of children being abused can be reduced are by:

- it being accepted as standard practice for staff to assist children to make their wishes and feelings known wherever possible;
- ensuring that children receive appropriate personal, health and social education (including sex education);
- ensuring that children know how to raise concerns, have access to a range of adults with whom they can communicate, and have a means of being heard available to them at all times.

(Department for Education and Skills 2006).

Children who need long-term respiratory support have the same right as other children to be protected from harm, and upholding this right is a vital part of working with them.

Summary

It is very likely that there will be times in your work with children who need long-term respiratory support when you feel that you want to question the ethics of a situation. Whilst there are often no easy answers to ethical dilemmas, the principles of beneficence, non-maleficence, autonomy and justice may help you to think about the various ethical aspects of the situation, and different people's views on this. You should also be mindful in your work of the obligations of veracity, fidelity, privacy and confidentiality.

Seeking informed consent should be a standard part of almost every aspect of your work. One of your responsibilities is to help children and families to achieve the greatest possible level of competence in decision-making and to support, but not coerce, them in the many decisions they have to make.

The children and families with whom you work have a number of rights, and you should aim to be aware of these, not only to ensure that you do not transgress them, but also so that you can assist those whom you support in having their rights met by society as a whole.

Chapter 13

Final notes

An increasing number of children require some form of long-term respiratory support, and it seems likely that the number of children who have this type of need will continue to rise. Wherever possible, the aim is for children and young people who need long-term respiratory support to be cared for at home, rather than in hospital, because their physical, emotional, social, educational and developmental needs will usually be better met in this familiar environment. However, whilst home care is generally the best option for children and their families, providing the day-to-day support that they need creates a number of challenges for all concerned.

The physical needs of a child or young person may only relate to their breathing, but some children have associated or separate physical problems, which you also have to know about. As well as needing to understand their individual physical needs, you may have to be able to work out how each problem is likely to affect and be affected by others. For example, if a child has chronic lung disease and gastro-oesophageal reflux, both problems may affect their breathing and feeding, and problems caused by one may worsen the problems caused by the other. In addition, where a child has a long-term respiratory problem, their exact needs, precisely how their breathing is affected, and how this is managed, are likely to be very individual. Many children do not conform to what the textbooks say, and it is often necessary to take the principles described, and work out how they have to be adapted, in order to meet the needs of the child or young person you care for.

Whilst it is the physical aspects of a child's needs that usually mean that their families need assistance, and it may seem as if these aspects of their care are difficult to learn about and complex to manage, other aspects of their support often present the greatest challenge. Working in someone else's home can be difficult for both staff and families. Whilst you are entitled to a satisfactory work environment, families are also seeking to establish and maintain a reasonable home life. Achieving both these outcomes can be problematic, and may require negotiation, and clarity about what should reasonably be expected by both parties.

Families generally very much need the support that you provide, but at the same time its necessity often intrudes on them and their lives. It can be difficult to achieve a balance between providing support that is effective and non-intrusive, and which acknowledges the parents' expertise in their child and their needs, while also providing meaningful assistance for them.

Understanding some of the challenges that the families of children who require long-term respiratory support are likely to face can be helpful in planning and providing effective support, which assists the child and family to maximise their life opportunities. It may be difficult for families to spend quality time together, in terms of having privacy at home and enjoying days out and holidays. A family's financial status is likely to be affected by their child having additional needs, because of changes in parents' employment status, and because of the additional expenses associated with the child's needs. This can impact on the whole family, the opportunities they have, and the stress they experience.

Children with a brother or sister who has additional needs may, in particular, be affected by their sibling's needs. Whilst providing care for siblings may be outside your direct remit, it can be helpful for you to be aware of the issues they may face, so that you can aim to tailor the provision for the child in question to minimise further disruption for the family. It may also be possible for you to note and highlight to their parents or service managers any ways in which the child's siblings might be helped.

Adolescents who need long-term respiratory support may face particular issues in relation to gaining the maximum possible level of independence, preparing for adult life and relationships, and in accessing education and employment. They may, whilst you are working with them, move from children's to adult services, and you may be well placed to assist in making this transition smooth and beneficial to them in the long term.

Children who need long-term respiratory support and their families are likely to feel loss related to their health needs. This may be because of their physical needs, the changes in their lives that these create, or the way in which they are provided for or viewed by society. Whilst you should not make any assumptions about what a child or members of their family see as a loss, it can be useful to consider what has changed or is different in their lives, and how this may affect them. This may help you to work with them sympathetically, and with greater understanding of the complexity of the feelings they may experience.

The provision of long-term respiratory support for children and young people brings with it a number of ethical and moral considerations. There are no easy answers to many such dilemmas, but it is useful for you to be aware of what they may include, and the different points of view that exist about them. These issues may relate to what is seen as being beneficial for children and families, what could be deemed to be harmful, and how limited resources can be fairly allocated. In all aspects of your work, you should consider how you can best maintain and promote the autonomy of children and their families, particularly in seeking to ascertain and act on children's views on everything that affects them.

All human beings have certain rights, and the rights of children and disabled people are legally protected. It is useful to know what these rights are, so that you can be certain that you maintain them yourself, encourage others to do so, and can advise those with whom you work about what reasonable expectations are.

Children who need long-term respiratory support are likely to have a fuller range of life experiences and opportunities if they are cared for at home, rather than in hospital. There are nonetheless many challenges to them having truly equal access to the range of life chances and experiences that their peers enjoy. One of your roles may be to assist them in gaining the greatest possible number of opportunities and advantages in their lives. This may include working with them, their families, schools, colleges and other parties to identify and encourage the achievement of maximum provision and inclusion, in a way that is meaningful and helpful to the child or young person concerned.

Although it may take time to feel confident in the knowledge and skills that are required to work with children who need long-term respiratory support, and their families, working with them in their homes can be very rewarding. Being aware of the range of issues that they may face should enable you to avoid problems and establish a useful, therapeutic and supportive relationship, with positive outcomes for the child and family. Whilst a child needing long-term respiratory support can create a significant workload and many disruptions for their family, the child is usually a much-loved and highly valued member of the family. The main focus of providing support should be to enable families to enjoy their relationship with their child, with all the rewards it brings, and to minimise the frustrations and difficulties created by the child's condition and provision for its trearment.

References

Abbott, D. and Howarth, J. (2007). Still off limits? Staff views on supporting gay, lesbian and bisexual people with learning disabilities to develop sexual and intimate relationships. *Journal of Applied Research in Intellectual Disabilities*, **20**(2): 116–26.

Abbott, D., Watson, D. and Townsley, R. (2005). The proof of the pudding: what difference does multi-agency working make to families with disabled children with complex healthcare needs? *Child and Family Social Work*, **10**(3): 229–38.

Allen, J. (2010). Pulmonary complications of neuromuscular disease: a respiratory mechanics perspective. *Paediatric Respiratory Review*, **11**(1): 18–23.

Appierto, L., Cori, M., Bianchi, R., Onofri, A., Catena, S., Ferrari, M. and Villani, A. (2002). Home care for chronic respiratory failure in children: 15 years experience. *Paediatric Anaesthesia*, **12**(4): 345–50.

Audit Commission (1993). *Children First: a study of hospital services*. HMSO. London.

Balfour-Lynn, I.M., Primhak, R.A. and Shaw, B.N.J. (2005). Home oxygen therapy for children: who, how and when. *Thorax* **60**(1): 78–81.

Balfour-Lynn, I.M., Field, D.J., Gringras, P., Hicks, B., Jardine, E., Jones, R.C., Magee, A.G., Primhak, R.A., Samuels, M.P., Shaw, N.J., Stevens, S., Sullivan, C., Taylor, J.A. and Wallis, C. (2009). *British Thoracic Society Guidelines for home oxygen in children. A quick reference guide*. British Thoracic Society. London.

Balling, K. and McCubbin, M. (2001). Hospitalized children with chronic illness: parental caregiving needs and valuing parental expertise. *Journal of Pediatric Nursing*, **16**(2): 110–19.

Barr, O. and Millar, R. (2003). Parents of children with intellectual disabilities: their expectations and experience of genetic counselling. *Journal of Applied Research in Intellectual Disabilities*, **16**(3): 189–204.

Bartlow, B. (2006). What, me grieve? Grieving and bereavement in daily dialysis practice. *Haemodialysis*, **10**(2): S46–S50.

Beauchamp, T.L. and Childress, J.F. (2001). *Principles of Biomedical Ethics*. Oxford University Press. Oxford.

Beresford, B. (2004) On the road to nowhere? Young disabled people and transition. *Child Care, Health and Development*, **30**(6): 581–87.

Bernard, C. (1999). Child sexual abuse and the black disabled child. *Disability and Society*, **14**(3): 325–40.

Berry, T. and Dawkins, B. (2004). *Don't Count Me Out*. MENCAP. London.

Boddy, J., Potts, P. and Stratham, J. (2006). *Models of good practice in joined-up assessment: working for children with 'significant and complex needs'*. Department for Education and Skills. London.

Booker, R. (2008). Pulse oximetry. *Nursing Standard*, **22**(30): 39–41.

Boosfeld, B. and O'Toole, M. (2000). Technology dependent children: from hospital to home. *Paediatric Nursing*, **12**(6): 20–22.

Brazier, M. (2006). *Critical care decisions in fetal and neonatal medicine: ethical issues*. Nuffield Council for Bioethics. London.

Breakey, W.J. (1997). Body image: the inner mirror. *Journal of Prosthetics and Orthotics*, **9**(3): 107–12.

Brett, J. (2004). The journey to accepting support: how parents of profoundly disabled children experience support in their lives. *Paediatric Nursing*, **16**(8): 14–18.

Buelow, J.M., McNelis, A., Shore, C.P. and Austin, J.K. (2006). Stressors of parents of children with epilepsy and intellectual disability. *Journal of Neurosciences Nursing*, **38**(3): 147–54, 176.

Burchardt, T. (2005). *The education and employment of disabled young people: frustrated ambition*. The Policy Press and Joseph Rowntree Foundation. Bristol.

Cambridge, P. (1999). The first hit: a case study of physical abuse of people with learning disabilities and challenging behaviour in a residential service. *Disability and Society*, **14**(3): 285–306.

Carnevale, F.A., Alexander, E., Davis, M., Renick, J. and Troini, R. (2006). Daily living with distress and enrichment: the moral experience of families with ventilator-assisted children at home. *Pediatrics*, **117**(1): 48–60.

Chamberlain, M.A. and Kent, R.M. (2005). The needs of young people with disabilities in the transition from paediatric to adult services. *Europa Medicophysica*, **41**(2): 111–23.

Christie, D. and Viner, R. (2005). Adolescent development. *British Medical Journal*, **330**(7486): 301–4.

Commission of Child Health Services (1976). *Fit for the Future (The Court Report)*. HMSO. London.

Contact a Family (2004a). *Relationships and caring for a disabled child.* Contact a Family. London.

Contact a Family (2004b). *Flexible enough?* Contact a Family. London.

Contact a Family (2005). *Grandparents*. Contact a Family. London.

Contact a Family (2007). *Siblings. Information for families*. Contact a Family. London.

Corden, A., Sloper, P. and Sainsbury, R. (2002). Financial effects for families after the death of a disabled or chronically ill child: a neglected dimension of bereavement. *Child Care, Health and Development*, **28**(3): 199–204.

Council of Europe (1950). European Convention on Human Rights. Convention for the Protection of Human Rights and Fundamental Freedoms, as amended by Protocol No. 11. Rome. Italy.

Davies, R. (2004). New understandings of parental grief: literature review. *Journal of Advanced Nursing*, **46**(5): 506–13.

Davies, S. and Hall, D. (2005). 'Contact a family' professionals and parents in partnership. *Archives of Diseases in Childhood*, **90**(10): 1053–57.

Dearden, C. and Becker, S. (2004). *Young Carers in the UK*. Carers UK and the Children's Society. London.

Department for Education and Skills and Department of Health (2006). *Transition: getting it right for young people*. DoH. London.

Department for Education and Skills (2006). *Working together to safeguard children: a guide to interagency working to safeguard and promote the welfare of children*. HMSO. London.

Department of Health (1989). *The Children Act*. HMSO. London.

Department of Health (2003). *Direct Payments Guidance: Community care, services for carers and children's services (Direct Payments) Guidance*. DoH, London.

Department of Health (2004a). *The National Service Framework for Children, Young People and Maternity Services*. DoH. London.

Department of Health (2004b). *The National Service Framework for Children, Young People and Maternity Services: disabled children and young people and those with complex health needs*. DoH. London.

Department of Health (2004c). *The Children Act*. HMSO. London.

Department of Health (2009). Individual budgets.
Available at http://webarchive.nationalarchives.gov.uk/+/www.dh.gov.uk/en/SocialCare/Socialcarereform/Personalisation/Individualbudgets/DH_089510

Department of Health (2011). Personal Health Budgets.
Available at http://www.dh.gov.uk/en/Healthcare/Personalhealthbudgets/index.htm

Dimond, B. (2005). Legal aspects of community care of the sick child. Chapter 12, pp.137–47, in Sidey, A. and Widdas, D. (eds) *Textbook of Community Children's Nursing*, second edition. Elsevier. London.

Donaldson, L. (2003). Expert patients usher in a new era of opportunity for the NHS. *British Medical Journal*, **326**(7402): 1279–80.

Donovan, M., Vanleit, B., Crowe, T.K. and Keefe, E. (2005). Occupational goals of mothers of children with disabilities. *American Journal of Occupational Therapy*, **59**(3): 249–61.

Draper, H. and Sorrell, T. (2002). Patients' responsibilities in medical ethics. *Bioethics*, **16**(4): 335–52.

Dyregrov, A. (2002). *Grief in Children*. Jessica Kingsley, London.

Eakes, G.G., Burke, M.L. and Hainsworth, M.A. (1998). Middle-range theory of chronic sorrow. *Journal of Nursing Scholarship*, **30**(2): 179–84.

Earle, S. (1999). Facilitated sex and the concept of sexual need: disabled students and their personal assistants. *Disability and Society*, **14**(3): 309–23.

Earle, S. (2001). Disability, facilitated sex and the role of the nurse. *Journal of Advanced Nursing*, **36**(3): 433–44.

European Court of Human Rights (2003). Convention for the Protection of Human Rights and Fundamental Freedoms, as amended by Protocol No. 11, Registry of the European Court of Human Rights.

Farasat, H. and Hewitt-Taylor, J. (2007). Learning to support children with complex and continuing health needs and their families. *Journal of Specialists in Pediatric Nursing*, **12**(2): 72–83.

Farnalls, S.L. and Rennick, J. (2003). Parents' caregiving approaches: facing a new treatment alternative in severe intractable childhood epilepsy. *Seizure*, **12**(1): 1–10.

Feldstein, S.W. and Miller, W.R. (2006). Substance use and risk taking amongst adolescents. *Journal of Mental Health*, **15**(6): 633–43.

Fletcher, L. and Buka, P. (1999). *A legal framework for caring*. Palgrave. Basingstoke.

Gillick Vs West Norfolk and Wisbeach Health Authority (1986). *Appeal Cases* 112–207.

Gilroy, C. and Johnson, P. (2004). Listening to the language of children's grief. *Groupwork*, **14**(3): 91–111.

Glendinning, C., Challis, D., Fernández, J.L., Jacobs, S., Jones, K., Knapp, M., Manthorpe, J., Moran, N., Netten, A., Stevens, M. and Wilberforce, M. (2008). *Evaluation of the Individual Budgets Pilot Programme Final Report*. York. IBSEN Social Policy Research Unit, University of York.

Godfrey, J. (1999). Empowerment through sexuality. pp. 172–86 in Wilkinson, G. and Miers, M. (eds) *Power and Nursing Practice*. Macmillan. London.

Grace, P.J. (2001). Professional advocacy: widening the scope of accountability. *Nursing Philosophy*, **2**(2): 151–62.

Greco, V., Sloper, P., Webb, R. and Beecham, J. (2006). Key worker services for disabled children: the views of staff. *Health and Social Care in the Community*. **14**(6): 445–52.

Green, S.E. (2001). Grandma's hands: parental perceptions of the importance of grandparents as secondary caregivers in families of children with disabilities. *International Journal of Ageing and Human Development*, **53**(1): 11–33.

Green, S.E. (2002). Mothering Amanda: musings on the experience of raising a child with cerebral palsy. *Journal of Loss and Trauma*, **7**(1): 21–34.

Green, S.E. (2007). 'We're tired, not sad': benefits and burdens of mothering a child with disability. *Social Science and Medicine*, **64**(1): 150–63.

Hall, E.O. (2004). A double concern: grandmothers' experiences when a small grandchild is critically ill. *Journal of Pediatric Nursing*, **19**(1): 61–69.

Hazel, R. (2006). The psychosocial impact on parents of tube feeding their child. *Paediatric Nursing*, **18**(4): 19–22.

Heaton, J. (2003). *Technology-dependent children and family life: research findings from the social policy research unit*. SPRU. University of York. York.

Heaton, J., Noyes, J., Sloper, P. and Shah, R. (2005). Families' experiences of caring for technology dependent children: a temporal perspective. *Health and Social Care in the Community*, **13**(5): 441–50.

Her Majesty's Stationery Office (1969). *The Family Law Reform Act*. HMSO. London.

Her Majesty's Stationery Office (1974). *The Health and Safety at Work Act*. HMSO. London.

Her Majesty's Stationery Office (1996). *Community Care Act (Direct Payments)*. HMSO. London.

Her Majesty's Stationery Office (1995). *The Disability Discrimination Act*. HMSO. London.

Her Majesty's Stationery Office (1998). *The Human Rights Act*. HMSO. London.

Her Majesty's Stationery Office (2000). *Carers and Disabled Children's Act*. HMSO. London.

Her Majesty's Stationery Office (2001). *The Special Educational Needs and Disability Act*. HMSO. London.

Her Majesty's Stationery Office (2005). *The Disability Discrimination Act*. HMSO. London.

Her Majesty's Stationery Office (2010) *The Equality Act*. HMSO. London.

Hewitt-Taylor, J. (2007). *Children with Complex and Continuing Health Needs*. Jessica Kingsley. London.

Hewitt-Taylor, J. (2008). Long-term mechanical ventilation part 2: principles. *British Journal of Healthcare Assistants*, **2**(9): 1–3.

Jaarsma, A.S., Knoester, H., van Rooyen, F. and Bos, A.P. (2001). Biphasic positive airway pressure ventilation (PeV+) in children. *Critical Care*, **5**(3): 174–77.

Joffe, S., Manocchia, M., Weeks, J.C. and Cleary, P.D. (2003). What do patients value in their hospital care? An empirical perspective on autonomy centered bioethics. *Journal of Medical Ethics*, **29**(2): 103–08.

Johnson, G. (2006). Confidentiality and standards of care. *Midwives*, **9**(12): 486–87.

Jubran, A. (1999). Pulse oximetry. *Critical Care*, **3**(2): R11–17.

Judson, L. (2004). Protective care: mothering a child dependent on parenteral nutrition. *Journal of Family Nursing*, **10**(1): 93–120.

Kaplan, C. (2002). Children and the law: The place of health professionals. *Child and Adolescent Mental Health*, **7**(4): 181–88.

Kearney, P. and Griffin, T. (2001). Between joy and sorrow: being a parent of a child with developmental disability. *Journal of Advanced Nursing*, **34**(5): 582–92.

Kennedy, I. (2003). Patients are experts in their own field. *British Medical Journal*, **326**(7402): 1276–77.

Kirk, S. and Glendinning, C. (2004). Developing services to support parents caring for a technology dependent child at home. *Child: Care, Health and Development*, **30**(3): 209–18.

Kirk, S., Glendinning, C. and Callery, P. (2005). Parent or nurse? the experience of being the parent of a technology dependent child. *Journal of Advanced Nursing*, **51**(5): 456–64.

Kirklin, D. (2007). Truth telling, autonomy and the role of metaphor. *Journal of Medical Ethics*, **33**(1): 11–14.

Koh, A. (1999). Non-judgemental care as a professional obligation. *Nursing Standard*, **13**(37): 38–41.

Kohler, M., Clarenbach, C.F., Boni, L., Brac, T., Russi, E.W. and Bloch, K.E. (2005). Quality of life, physical disability, and respiratory impairment in Duchenne Muscular Dystrophy. *American Journal of Respiratory and Critical Care Medicine*, **172**(8): 1032–36.

Krueger, G. (2006). Meaning making in the aftermath of sudden infant death syndrome. *Nursing Inquiry*, **13**(3): 163–71.

Kübler Ross, E. (1969). *On Death and Dying*. Macmillan. New York.

Kübler Ross, E. (1997). *On Death and Dying*. Touchstone. New York.

Landsman, G.H. (1998). Reconstructing motherhood in the age of 'perfect babies': Mothers of infants and toddlers with disabilities. *Signs*, **24**(1): 69–99.

Landsman, G. (2005) Mothers and models of disability. *Journal of Medical Humanities*, **26**(2/3): 121–39.

Lassetter, J.H., Mandleco, B.L. and Roper, S.O. (2007). Family photographs: expressions of parents raising children with disabilities. *Qualitative Health Research*, **17**(4): 456–567.

Levine, C. (2005). Acceptance, avoidance, and ambiguity: conflicting social values about childhood disability. *Kennedy Institute of Ethics Journal*, **15**(4): 371–83.

Lowden, J. (2002). Children's rights: a decade of dispute. *Journal of Advanced Nursing*, **37**(1): 100–07.

Lynes, D. and Kelly, C. (2009). Domiciliary oxygen therapy: assessment and management. *Nursing Standard*, **23**(20): 50–56.

MacDonald, H. and Callery, P. (2004) Different meanings of respite: a study of parents, nurses and social workers caring for children with complex needs. *Child: Care, Health and Development*, **30**(3): 279–88.

MacGregor, J. (2008). *Introduction to the Anatomy and Physiology of Children*, second edition. Routledge. London and New York.

Marcus, C.L., Rosen, G., Davidson Ward, S.L., Halblower, A.C., Sterni, L., Lutz, J., Standing, P.J., Bolduc, D. and Gordon, N. (2006). Adherence to and effectiveness of positive airway pressure therapy in children with obstructive sleep apnea. *Pediatrics*, **117**(3): e442–51.

Margolan, H., Fraser, J. and Lenton, S. (2004). Parental experiences of services when their child requires long-term ventilation. Implications for commissioning and providing services. *Child: Care, Health and Development*, **30**(3): 257–64.

McCann, E. (2000). The expression of sexuality in people with psychosis: breaking the taboos. *Journal of Advanced Nursing*, **32**(1): 132–38.

McClure, L. (2005). Young carers and community children's nursing, Chapter 26, pp. 289–97, in Sidey, A. and Widdas, D. (eds). *Textbook of Community Children's Nursing*, second edition. Elsevier. London.

McConkey, R. and Smyth, M. (2003). Parental perceptions of risks with older teenagers who have severe learning difficulties contrasted with the young people's views and experiences. *Children and Society*, **17**(1): 18–31.

McGloin, S. (2008). Administration of oxygen therapy. *Nursing Standard*, **21**(22): 46–48.

McLelland, R. (2006). *European Standards on Confidentiality and Privacy in Healthcare*. Queen's University, Belfast.

Meehan, D.R. (2005). Mothering a 3- to 6-year-old child with hemiparesis. *Journal of Neurosciences Nursing*, **37**(5): 265–71.

Menahem, S. and Grimwade, J. (2003). Pregnancy termination following prenatal diagnosis of serious heart disease in the fetus. *Early Human Development*, **73**(1): 71–78.

Millar, S. and Aitken, S. (2005). *FE and Complex Needs. Views of children and young people*. Communication Aids for Language and Learning Centre, University of Edinburgh, Edinburgh.

Miller, A.R., Condin, C.J., McKellin, W.H., Shaw, S., Klassen, A.F. and Sheps, S. (2009). *Continuity of care for children with complex chronic health conditions: parents' perspectives*. BMC Health Services Research. 9:242 doi: 10.1186/1472-6963-9-242.

Mok, Y.S. (2005). Respect based toleration. *Nursing Philosophy*, **6**(4): 274–77.

Morton, P., Fontaine, D.K., Hudat, C.M. and Gallo, B.M. (2005). *Critical Care Nursing*, eighth edition. Lippincott-Williams. Philadelphia.

Mulligan, S. (2003). *Occupational Therapy Evaluation for Children: A pocket guide*. Lippincott Williams & Wilkins. Baltimore.

Nessa, N. (2004). *The Health of Children and Young People: Disability*. Office for National Statistics. London.

Neufeld, S.M., Query, B. and Drummond, J.E. (2001). Respite care users who have children with chronic conditions: are they getting a break? *Journal of Pediatric Nursing*, **16**(4): 234–44.

NHS Quality Improvement Scotland (2008). *Caring for the Child/Young Person with a Tracheostomy*. Edinburgh. NHS Quality Improvement Scotland.

Nicolai, T. (2006). The physiological basis of respiratory support. *Paediatric Respiratory Reviews*, **7**(2): 97–102.

Noyes, J. (2006). Health and quality of life of ventilator-dependent children. *Journal of Advanced Nursing*, **56**(4): 392–403.

Noyes, J., Godfrey, C. and Beecham, J. (2006). Resource use and service costs for ventilator-dependent children and young people in the UK. *Health and Social Care in the Community*. **14**(6): 508–22.

Nursing and Midwifery Council (2008). *The code: Standards of conduct, performance and ethics for nurses and midwives*. London, Nursing and Midwifery Council.

Nuutila, L. and Salantera, S. (2005). Children with long-term illness: parents' experiences of care. *Journal of Pediatric Nursing*, **21**(2): 153–60.

Nye, R.A. (1999). *Sexuality*. Oxford University Press. Oxford.

O'Brien, M.E. and Wegner, C.B. (2002). Rearing the child who is technology dependent: perceptions of parents and home care nurses. *Journal of Specialist Pediatric Nursing*, **7**(1): 7–15.

Office of the United Nations High Commissioner for Human Rights (1989). *The United Nations Convention on the Rights of the Child*. Office of the United Nations High Commissioner for Human Rights. Geneva. Switzerland.

OFSTED (2004). Special education needs and disability: towards inclusive schools. HMI 2276. OFSTED. Manchester.http://www.ofsted.gov.uk/Ofsted-home/Publications-and-research/Browse-all-by/Documents-by-type/Thematic-reports/Special-educational-needs-and-disability-towards-inclusive-schools/(language)/eng-GB
Accessed November 19th 2010

OFSTED (2010). *The Special Education Needs and Disability Review*. OFSTED. Manchester.

Olsen, D.P., Dixon, J.K., Grey, M., Deshefy-Longhi, T. and Demarest, J.C. (2005). Privacy concerns of patients and nurse practitioners in primary care. *Journal of the American Academy of Nurse Practitioners*, **17**(12): 527–34.

Orfali, K. and Gordon, E. (2004). Autonomy gone awry: a cross-cultural study of parents' experiences in neonatal intensive care units. *Theoretical Medicine and Bioethics*, **25**(4): 329–65.

Paragas, J. (2008). Keeping the beat with pulse oximetry. *Nursing*, **38**(11): 56hn1–56hn2.

Parekh, S.A. (2006). Child consent and the law: an insight and discussion into the law relating to consent and competence. *Child: Health, Care and Development*, **33**(1): 78–82.

Parker, G., Bhakta, P., Lovett, C., Olsen, R., Paisley, S. and Turner, D. (2006). Paediatric home care: a systematic reviews of randomized trials on costs and effectiveness. *Journal of Health Service Research Policy*, **11**(2): 110–19.

Parkes, C.M. and Markus, A. (eds). (1998). *Coping with Loss: Helping Patients and their Families*. BMJ Books. London.

Philip, A.G.S. (2009). Chronic lung disease of prematurity: a short history. *Seminars in Fetal and Neonatal Medicine*, **14**(6): 333–38.

Pierce, D. and Marshall, A. (2004). Maternal management of home space and time to facilitate infant/toddlers play and development. Chapter 4, pp. 73–94, in Esdaile, S.A. and Olson, J.A. (eds) *Mothering Occupations: Challenge, Agency and Participation*. FA Davis Co. Philadelphia.

Platt, H. (1959). *The Welfare of Children in Hospital (report of the committee)*. Ministry of Health commissioned report. Central Health Services. London.

Poses, R.M. (2003). A cautionary tale: the dysfunction of American healthcare. *European Journal of Internal Medicine*, **14**(2): 123–30.

Potgieter, C.A. and Gadij, K. (2005). Sexual self-esteem and body image of South African spinal cord injured adolescents. *Sexuality and Disability*, **23**(1) 1–20.

Redmond, B. and Richardson, V. (2003). Just getting on with it: exploring the service needs of mothers who care for young children with severe/profound and life threatening intellectual disability. *Journal of Applied Research in Intellectual Disabilities*, **16**(4): 205–18.

Rehm, R.S. and Bradley, J.F. (2005). Normalization in families raising a child who is medically fragile/technology dependent and developmentally delayed. *Qualitative Health Research*, **15**(6): 807–20.

Reyna, V.F. and Farley, F. (2006). Risk and rationality in adolescent decision making: implications for theory, practice, and public policy. *Psychological Science in the Public Interest*, **7**(1): 1–44.

Riesz, E. (2004). Loss and transitions: A 30-year perspective on life with a child who has Downs Syndrome. *Journal of Loss and Trauma*, **9**(4): 371–82.

Riley, M. (2003). Facilitating children's grief. *Journal of School Nursing*, **19**(4): 212–18.

Ronayne, S. (2001). Nurse-patient partnerships in hospital care. *Journal of Clinical Nursing*, **10**(5): 591–92.

Rosenblatt, P.C. (2000). *Parent Grief: Narratives of Loss and Relationship*. Brunner-Mazl Inc. Philadelphia.

Rowse, V. (2007). Consent in severely disabled children: informed or an infringement of their human rights. *Journal of Child Healthcare*, **11**(1): 70–77.

Royal College of Nursing (2003). *Defining Nursing*. Royal College of Nursing. London.

Russell, P. (2003). Access and achievement or social exclusion? Are the government's policies working for disabled children and their families? *Children and Society*, **17**(3): 215–25.

Sakellariou, D. and Algado, S.S. (2006). Sexuality and disability: a case of occupational injustice. *British Journal of Occupational Therapy*, **69**(2): 69–76.

Saladin, K.S. and Miller, L. (2004). *Anatomy and Physiology: the unity of form and function*, third edition. London and Boston, McGraw-Hill.

Saldinger, A., Cain, A., Kalter, N. and Iohnes, K. (1999). Anticipating parental death in families with children. *American Journal of Orthopsychiatry*, **69**(1): 39–47.

Samwell, B. (2005). Nursing the family and supporting the nurse. Chapter 11, pp. 129–36, in Sidey, A. and Widdas, D. (eds) *Textbook of Community Children's Nursing*, second edition. Elsevier. London.

Sant Angelo, D. (2000). Learning disability community nursing. Addressing emotional and sexual health needs. Chapter 4. pp. 52–68, in Astor, R. and Jeffries, K. (eds) *Positive Initiatives for People with Learning Difficulties: Promoting Healthy Lifestyles*. Macmillan Press. Basingstoke.

Scorgie, K. and Sobsey, D. (2000). Transformational outcomes associated with parenting children who have disabilities. *Mental Retardation*, **38**(3): 195–206.

Scornaienchi, J.M. (2003). Chronic sorrow: one mother's experience with two children with lissencephaly. *Journal of Paediatric Healthcare*, **17**(6): 290–94.

Scourfield, P. (2005). Implementing the Community Care (Direct Payments) Act: Will the supply of personal assistants meet the demand and at what price? *Journal of Social Policy*, **34**(3): 469–88.

Serwint, J. (2004). One method of coping: resident debriefing after the death of a patient. *Journal of Pediatrics*, **145**(2): 229–34.

Shakespeare, T. (1999). The sexual politics of disabled masculinity. *Sexuality and Disability*, **17**(1): 53–64.

Sharland, E. (2006). *Young People, Risk Taking and Risk Making: Some Thoughts for Social Work*. Forum Qualitative Sozialforschung/ Forum:Qualitative Social Research 7(1), Art. 23. http://www.qualitative-research.net/index.php/fqs/article/view/56/116 Accessed 19/10/10.

Sharpe, D. and Rossiter, L. (2002). Siblings of children with a chronic illness: A meta-analysis. *Journal of Pediatric Psychology*, **27**(8): 699–710.

Shribman, S. (2007). *Making it Better: For Children and Young People*. Department of Health. London.

Singh, I. (2005). *Anatomy and Physiology for Nurses*. Anshan. Tunbridge Wells.

Skar, L. (2002). Disabled children's perceptions of technical aids, assistance and peers in play situations. *Scandinavian Journal of Caring Sciences*, **16**(1): 27–33.

Sly, D.P. and Collins, R.A. (2006). Physiological basis of respiratory signs and symptoms. *Paediatric Respiratory Reviews*, **7**(2): 84–88.

Smith, L.J., McKay, K.O., Van Asperen, P.P., Selvadurai, H. and Fitzgerald, D.A. (2010). Normal development of the lung and premature birth. *Paediatric Respiratory Reviews*, **11**(3): 135–42.

Soanes, C., Waite, M. and Hawker, S. (2001). *Oxford Dictionary and Thesaurus*. Oxford University Press. Oxford.

Steinberg, L. (2007). Risk taking in adolescence. New perspectives from brain and behavioural science. *Current Directions in Psychological Science*, **16**(2): 55–59.

Stipek, D., Recchia, S. and McClintic, S. (1992). Self-evaluation in young children. *Monographs of the Society for Research in Child Development*, **57**(1): 1–98.

Strandmark, M.K. (2004). Ill health is powerlessness: a phenomenological study about worthlessness, limitations and suffering. *Scandinavian Journal of Caring Sciences*, **18**(2): 135–44.

Sturgess, J. (2003). A model describing play as a child-chosen activity: is this still valid in contemporary Australia? *Australian Occupational Therapy Journal*, **50**(2): 104–08.

Sullivan, M. (2003). The new subjective medicine: taking the patient's point of view on healthcare and health. *Social Science and Medicine*, **56**(7): 1595–604.

Sussenberger, B. (2003). Socioeconomic factors and their influence on occupational performance. Chapter 8, pp. 97–110, in Crepeau, E., Cohn, E. and Schell, B. (eds.) *Willard and Spackman's Occupational Therapy,* tenth edition. Lippincott, Williams & Wilkins. Philadelphia.

Sweet, D.G. and Halliday H.L. (2002). Airway remodelling in chronic lung disease of prematurity. *Paediatric Respiratory Reviews*, **3**(2): 140–46.

Taylor, B. and Donnelly, M. (2006). Risks to home care workers: professional perspectives. *Health, Risk and Society*, **8**(3): 239–56.

Taylor, V., Fuggle, P. and Charman, T. (2001). Well sibling psychological adjustment to chronic physical disorder in a sibling: how important is maternal awareness of their illness attitudes and perceptions? *Journal of Child Psychology and Psychiatry*, **42**(7): 953–62.

Thornton, P. (2003). *What Works and Looking Ahead: UK Policies and Practices Facilitating Employment of Disabled People*. Social Policy Research Unit. University of York. York.

Thurston, S., Paul, L., Ye, C., Loney, P., Browne, G., Thabane, L. and Rosenbaum, P. (2010). Interactions among ecological factors that explain the psychosocial quality of life of children with complex needs. *International Journal of Pediatrics*, vol. 2010, Article ID 404687, 10 pages, 2010. doi:10.1155/2010/404687

Available at http://www.hindawi.com/journals/ijped/2010/404687.html Accessed 19/11/10.

Todd, S. and Jones, S. (2005). Looking at the future and seeing the past: the challenge of the middle years of parenting a child with intellectual disabilities. *Journal of Intellectual Disability Research*, **49**(6): 389–404.

Tuckett, A.G. (1998). Code of ethics: assistance with a lie choice? *Australian Journal of Holistic Nursing*, **5**(2): 36–40.

Turner, C. (2006). Fact Sheet 38. *Adolescents with Tuberous Sclerosis Complex*. Tuberous Sclerosis Association. Birmingham.

Valdez-Lowe, C., Ghareeb, S.A. and Artinian, N.T. (2009) Pulse oximetry in adults. *American Journal of Nursing*, **109**(6): 52–59.

Walter, T. (1996). A new model of grief: bereavement and biography. *Mortality*, **1**(1): 7–25.

Wang, K.K. and Barnard, A. (2004). Technology dependent children and their families: a review. *Journal of Advanced Nursing*, **45**(1): 36–46.

Watson, D., Abbott, D. and Townsley, R. (2006). Listen to me too! Lessons from involving children with complex healthcare needs in research about multi-agency services. *Child: Care, Health and Development*, **33**(1): 90–95.

Weese-Mayer, D.E., Berry-Kravis, E.M., Ceccherini, I., Keens, T.G., Loghmanee, D.A. and Trang, H. (2010). ATS Congenital Central Hypoventilation Syndrome Subcommittee. An official ATS clinical policy statement: Congenital central hypoventilation syndrome: genetic basis, diagnosis, and management. *American Journal of Respiratory Critical Care Medicine*, **181**(6): 626–44.

Whitehurst, T. (2006). Liberating silent voices – perspectives of children with profound and complex learning needs on inclusion. *British Journal of Learning Disabilities*, **35**(1): 55–61.

Widdas, D., Sidey, A. and Dryden, S. (2005) Delivering and funding care for children with complex needs. Chapter 22, pp. 249–60, in Sidey, A. and Widdas, D. (eds) *Textbook of Community Children's Nursing*, second edition. Elsevier. London.

Williams, C. and Asquith, J. (2000). *Paediatric Intensive Care*. Churchill Livingstone. London.

Wilmot, S. (2003). *Ethics, Power and Policy: the Future of Nursing in the NHS*. Palgrave. Basingstoke.

Wolfson, L. (2004) Family well being and disabled children: a psychosocial model of disability-related child behaviour problems. *British Journal of Health Psychology*, **9**(1): 1–13.

Wood, J.D. and Milo, E. (2001). Father's grief when a disabled child dies. *Death Studies*, **25**(8): 635–61.

Woodrow, P. (2005). *Intensive Care Nursing*, second edition. London, Routledge.

Worden, J.W. (1991). *Grief Counselling and Grief Therapy*. Springer. New York.

Yantzi, N.M., Rosenberg, M.W. and McKeever, P. (2006). Getting out of the house: the challenges mothers face when their children have long term care needs. *Health and Social Care in the Community*, **15**(1): 45–55.

Zijlstra, H.P. and Vlaskamp, C. (2005). The impact of medical conditions on the support of children with profound intellectual and multiple disabilities. *Journal of Applied Research in Intellectual Disabilities*, **18**(2): 151–61.

Index

Coventry University Library